A COLOUR ATLAS OF
DERMATOLOGY

D1356410

Copyright © G M Levene & C D Calnan, 1974
Published by Wolfe Medical Publications Ltd, 1974
Printed by Smeets-Weert, Holland
ISBN 0 7234 0174 8
10th impression 1984

General Editor, Wolfe Medical Books
G Barry Carruthers MD (Lond)

This book is one of the titles in the series of
Wolfe Medical Atlases, a series which brings together
probably the world's largest systematic published
collection of diagnostic colour photographs.
   For a full list of Atlases in the series, plus
forthcoming titles and details of our surgical, dental
and veterinary Atlases, please write to
Wolfe Medical Publications Ltd, Wolfe House,
3 Conway Street, London W1P 6HE.

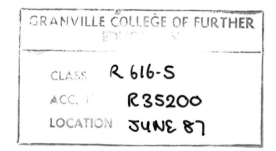

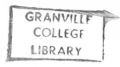
A colour atlas
of
Dermatology

G. M. LEVENE
MB, MRCP
*Consultant Dermatologist, St John's Hospital for
Diseases of the Skin, London
Consultant Dermatologist, Middlesex Hospital, London*

&

C. D. CALNAN
MA, MB, B Chir, FRCP
*Consultant Dermatologist, St John's Hospital for
Diseases of the Skin
and The Royal Free Hospital, London*

WOLFE MEDICAL PUBLICATIONS LTD

ACKNOWLEDGEMENTS

We wish to thank Dr R H Meara, Dean of The Institute of Dermatology and the Consultant Staff of St John's Hospital for Diseases of the Skin, London, for access to their collection of photographs. It is also a pleasure to acknowledge the help given by Mr R R Phillips, Director of the Department of Medical Illustration of the Institute, and his Staff. We are indebted to Dr H J Wallace and Dr G C Wells of St Thomas's Hospital for constant encouragement during the earliest stages of this work. For providing one or more individual photographs we are most grateful to Dr E Abell, Dr Yvonne Clayton, Dr C A Ramsay and Dr I Sarkany.

Figure **95** is from 'A Colour Atlas of Oro-Facial Diseases' by Mr L W Kay and Mr R Haskell. Figures **128**, **147** and **178** are from 'A Colour Atlas of Venereology' by Dr Anthony Wisdom.

Messrs Faber and Faber have kindly allowed us to reproduce the skin diagram which appears on page 10 in this volume. It previously appeared in 'A General Textbook of Nursing', 18th edition, by Evelyn Pearce.

To S.L. and H.L.

CONTENTS

PREFACE

Clinical dermatology is a subject in which entities tend to be well-marked and diagnosable with some precision by skilled inspection. This atlas has been prepared to help medical students, practitioners and those starting training in dermatology to become acquainted with the distinctive features of skin diseases. Most common disorders are illustrated and also several rare ones which are important with regard to associated systemic disease or to differential diagnosis. Teachers may find it useful to demonstrate features of lesions to students in their clinics.

The emphasis throughout is on diagnosis and differential diagnosis and, to facilitate this, cross-references are provided in the captions, in the introductions to sections, and in the index.

Eighty-five per cent of the photographs in this atlas were taken by the first author using a Kodak Retina Reflex III camera and Kodachrome film. The light source was a single Metz '180' flash unit. The selection of photographs necessarily reflects experience of dermatological practice in London but we believe that the range of disorders included will be helpful to practitioners in whichever community they are working.

INTRODUCTION

Modern techniques in histopathology, mycology, biochemistry, immunology and photobiology are constantly improving the accuracy of diagnosis and are expanding our understanding of the basic mechanisms of cutaneous disease. Their importance cannot be overemphasized, however at the present time it remains true that the single most useful procedure which will influence the management of patients is the visual inspection of their lesions.

It is necessary for the student to become reasonably fluent in the terms used specifically to describe skin lesions. The commonest terms are defined on pages 10–15 and some of them are illustrated by line drawings. The diagram of the vertical section of skin on page 10 shows the structural features which are referred to throughout the book. The position of pigment cells (not shown in the diagram) is described briefly on page 186.

Dermatology is particularly rich in synonyms in the nomenclature of diseases. It is best to regard many disease designations simply as code names employed to convey the concept of a pathological entity. The choice of titles used here reflects current usage in the United Kingdom. Where a title seems especially liable to mislead inverted commas are used (e.g. 'seborrhoeic' dermatitis, 'toxic' erythema).

Accurate history taking must not be neglected and should include details of the duration of the eruption, its site and mode of onset, its fluctuations with and without treatment, any skin trouble in the past, whether other members of the family or cohabitants are affected, and the presence or absence of itching and pain. Further questions will suggest themselves as the patient is examined.

If mistakes or omissions are to be avoided it will often be necessary to examine the whole of the skin surface (and mouth) in a good light, preferably daylight. The findings should be recorded in terms of (*a*) the morphology of individual lesions, (*b*) the distribution of lesions and (*c*) the arrangement or grouping of lesions. From this information diagnostic possibilities can be considered in order of probability and the need for special investigations assessed.

COMMON TERMS IN DERMATOLOGY

Dermatology, like any other speciality, has its own group of descriptive technical terms. Fortunately these are few and easily remembered.

HAIRS

OPENINGS
OF SWEAT
GLANDS

EPIDERMIS

HORNY
LAYER

GRANULAR
LAYER

PRICKLE-CELL
LAYER

BASAL
LAYER

SKIN

BLOOD
VESSELS

DERMIS

HAIR
FOLLICLE

NERVES

SUBCUTANEOUS FATTY TISSUE

diagram of skin structure

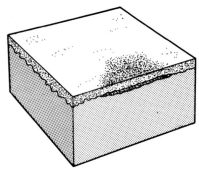

Macule A flat spot or patch of a different colour from the surrounding skin, e.g. freckles.

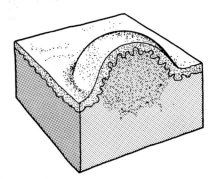

Papule A raised spot on the surface of the skin, e.g. lichen planus.

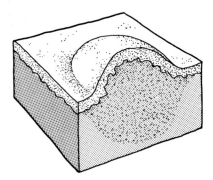

Nodule Usually indicates a lump deeply set in the skin, e.g. calcinosis.

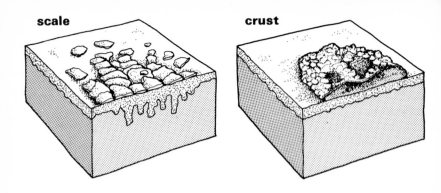

Scale A flake of flat horny cells loosened from the horny layer (stratum corneum), e.g. psoriasis.

Crust Usually refers to dried serum (serous crust), but sometimes the term is applied to a thick mass of horny cells (keratin crust) or to a mixture of both.

Pustule A skin bleb filled with pus.

Cyst A deeply situated fluid-filled cavity.

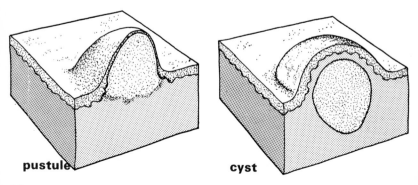

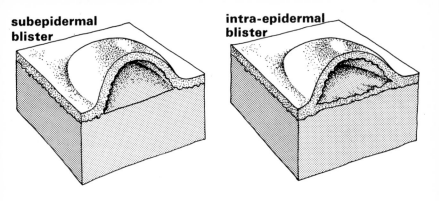

subepidermal blister

intra-epidermal blister

Blister A skin bleb filled with clear fluid. It may be :

   subepidermal, e.g. pemphigoid and dermatitis herpetiformis.

   intra-epidermal, e.g. pemphigus, eczema.

   subcorneal, e.g. impetigo.

Fissure A crack or split in the epidermis.

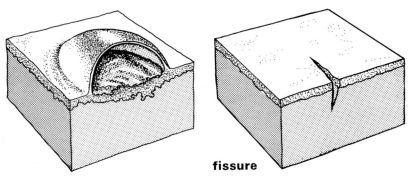

fissure

subcorneal blister

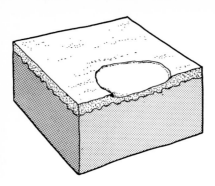

Erosion An area of partial loss of epithelium of skin or mucous membrane.

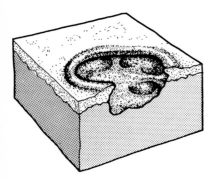

Ulcer An area of total loss of epithelium of skin or mucous membrane.

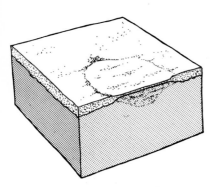

Atrophy Loss of thickness or substance of the epidermis, dermis or other tissue.

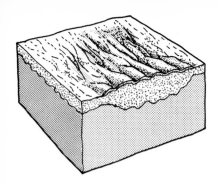

Lichenification Thickening of both the prickle-cell layer and horny layer of the epidermis with underlying inflammation giving the skin a mauvish 'morocco leather' appearance with exaggeration of normal skin lines seen in relief, e.g. lichen simplex.

Not illustrated

Vesicle A small blister, e.g. herpes simplex, eczema.

Excoriation A scratch mark which has scored the epidermis.

Plaque A raised uniform thickening of a portion of the skin with a well-defined edge and a flat or rough surface, e.g. psoriasis.

Erythema *adj.* redness ; *noun*, an eruption with dilatation of dermal blood vessels and oedema, e.g. 'toxic' erythema.

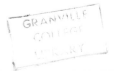

PSORIASIS

Psoriasis is a disorder in which there is loss of control of normal epidermal cell turnover. Increased mitosis of epidermal cells results in thickening of the epidermis and the production of imperfect keratin scales. Associated with the epidermal changes are dermal vasodilatation, oedema and infiltration with polymorphonuclear leucocytes. It is not known what causes the localised disturbance of epidermal control.

1 *Psoriasis, elbows* Lesions are sharply circumscribed bright red plaques covered with coarse silvery scales. The elbows and knees are commonly involved and lesions are usually symmetrically distributed.

The cause of psoriasis is unknown. A family history of the condition is obtained in about a third of cases. Most cases begin in the second and third decade of life. It is rare below the age of five. Its course is unpredictable and lesions are usually present to a greater or lesser extent throughout life.

2 *Psoriasis* Typical small plaques showing exfoliation of silvery scales after gentle scraping with a spatula or fingernail. This is a helpful diagnostic procedure.

3 *Psoriasis, elbows* Partial treatment with ointment has cleared the scales, leaving erythematous plaques.

1

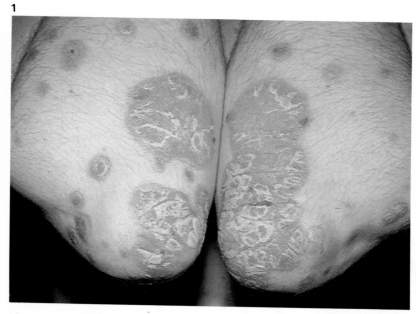

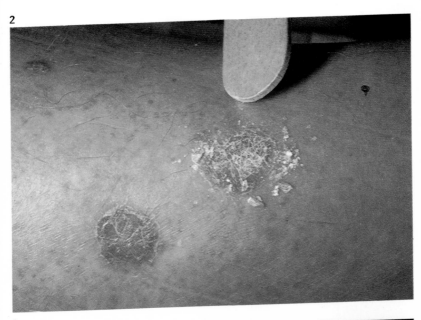

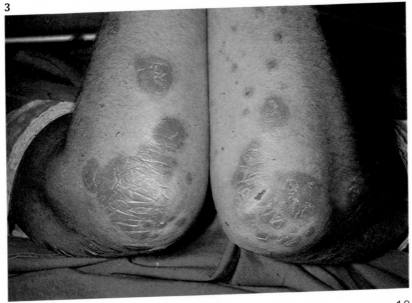

4 *Psoriasis, knees* A thick layer of keratin is obscuring underlying erythema.

5 *Psoriasis, lumbar* An extensive chronic plaque of thickened psoriasis is often found in this area.

6 *Psoriasis, Köbner phenomenon* The term 'Köbner phenomenon' means the development of a skin disease at the site of minor trauma when it is already active on other parts of the skin. This example was caused by a tight brassière and the line of psoriasis under the shoulder strap is clearly seen. Other skin diseases which are often reproduced at sites of trauma are viral warts (**142**), molluscum contagiosum (**148**) and lichen planus (**188**).

4

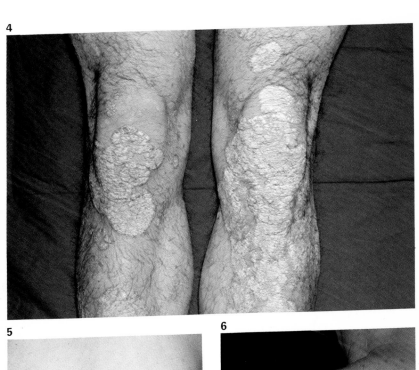

5

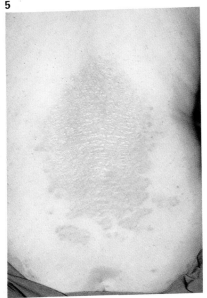

6

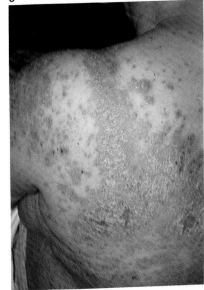

7 *Psoriasis, trunk, annular* Often plaques will heal centrally and continue to spread peripherally giving an annular configuration. Many skin diseases typically or exceptionally produce annular or arcuate lesions (see Index, 'Annular and arcuate lesions') so that this configuration is of only limited help in diagnosis.

8 *Psoriasis, flexural, perineum* Perineal, submammary and axillary psoriasis is pink, moist and glazed with minimal or absent scaling. In these situations it can be confused with candidal infection, fungal infection and other types of intertrigo. Helpful points in diagnosis are the sharply circumscribed margins of the erythema and the presence of typical psoriatic lesions elsewhere.

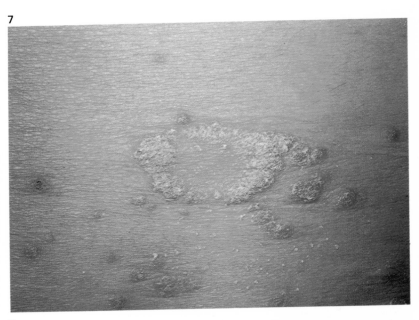

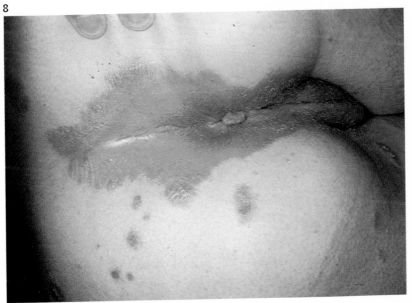

9 *Psoriasis, scalp and hair margin*   The scalp is commonly affected and the presence of coarse white or yellowish-white scales in palpable plaques gives the diagnosis. There is often a tendency, as here, for the plaques to spread out beyond the hair margin. The presence of normal scalp skin between plaques distinguishes psoriasis from dandruff (pityriasis capitis) and seborrhoeic dermatitis. Visible loss of hair in psoriatic scalp plaques is uncommon.

10 *Psoriasis, nails*   The fingernails show coarse 'thimble' pitting which is pathognomonic. All three nails show areas with regular pits, some of them in longitudinal formation. Nail dystrophy may be the only evidence of psoriasis.

9

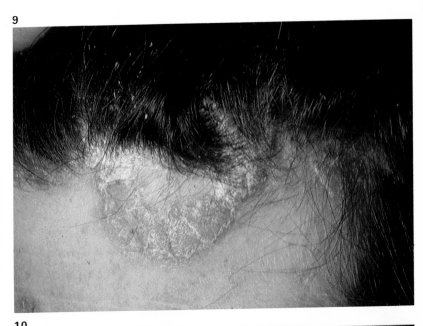

10

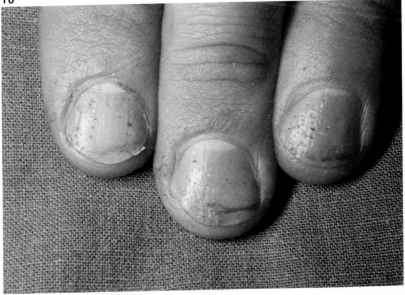

11 *Psoriasis, fingernails* The distal separation of the nail plate (onycholysis) and the irregular salmon-coloured patch are typical of psoriasis.

12 *Psoriasis, penis* A common site. In the uncircumcised the appearance is that of flexural psoriasis.

13 *Psoriasis, palms* Hard dome-shaped lesions are present. It is important to look for psoriasis elsewhere on the skin. Secondary syphilis can look similar to this (**93**).

11

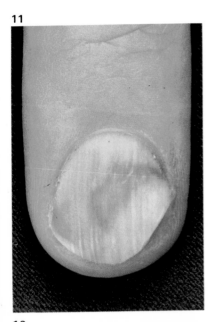

12

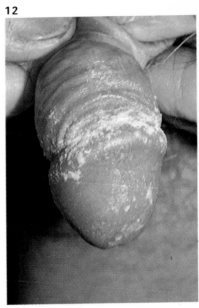

13

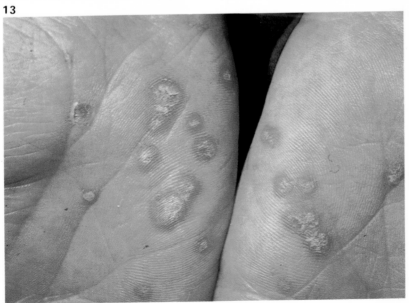

14 *Psoriasis, guttate* The 'spattered' droplet type of psoriasis occurs especially in children and young adults usually following a strepto-coccal throat infection. There is no predilection for the elbows and knees. It usually clears completely in a few months when the infection resolves, but classical psoriasis may develop subsequently.

15 *Psoriasis, erythrodermic* Starting as typical common psoriasis it spreads to involve the whole skin surface. This is one type of erythro-derma (formerly called exfoliative dermatitis), of which there are other causes such as eczema (**70**), reticulosis (**449**) and pityriasis rubra pilaris (**246**).

16 *Psoriasis with psoriatic arthropathy, finger* Psoriatic arthro-pathy resembles rheumatoid arthritis, but serum rheumatoid factor is absent. Distal interphalangeal joint arthritis is characteristic but is by no means always present. Pain and swelling of the finger joints and large joints of the limbs is present in between 5% and 10% of patients with psoriasis and can result in severe disability.

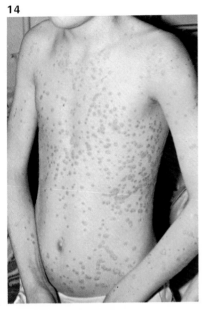

14

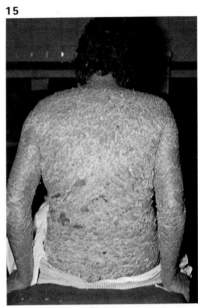

15

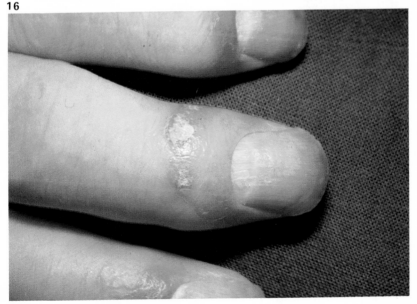

16

17 *Psoriasis, pustular, palms* The commonest presentation of pustular psoriasis is localised to the palms and soles with no evidence of psoriasis elsewhere. Old pustules leave brownish stains and new ones appear. Sometimes it is part of a generalised pustular psoriasis (**20**). The pus is sterile and this together with the absence of severe tenderness and oedema distinguishes it from infected acute eczema of the palms (**66**).

18 *Psoriasis, pustular, soles* The same observations apply as for the palmar variety. Usually both palms and soles are affected but not always to the same degree.

19 *Psoriasis, pustular, fingertips* Formerly called 'acrodermatitis continua of Hallopeau', this paronychial type affects the extremities of the fingers and toes and may extend proximally. Rarely it may progress to generalised pustular psoriasis with a bad prognosis. The nails tend to be shed at an early stage.

17

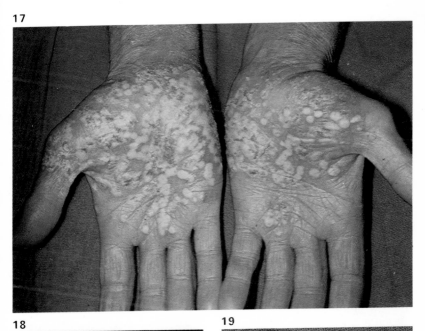

18

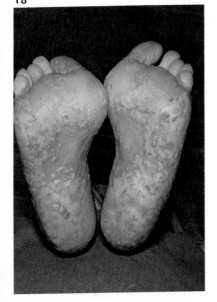

19

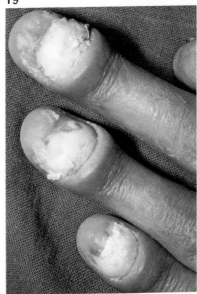

20 *Generalised pustular psoriasis (von Zumbusch)* The patient is severely ill with high fever and prostration. A polymorph leukocytosis of up to 30,000 is present, and there is low serum calcium and steatorrhoea. Widespread crops of superficial pustules appear from day to day on a bright red background. It can be precipitated by systemic corticosteriods. Untreated, this form of psoriasis is not infrequently fatal. When it appears during pregnancy it has been called 'impetigo herpetiformis'.

21 *Psoriasis, tongue* This very rare phenomenon occurs only in generalised pustular psoriasis. Its severity varies in direct proportion to the skin lesions. The appearance is similar to that of 'geographical tongue' (**275**).

20

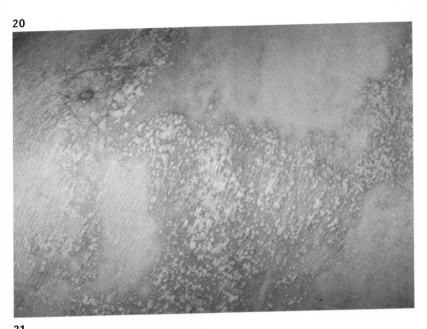

21

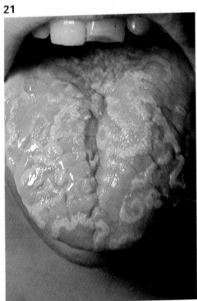

DERMATITIS/ECZEMA

The terms dermatitis and eczema are best regarded as synonymous. To emphasize this point the designation dermatitis/eczema will often appear although normally only one word is used. It refers to a type of inflammation of the skin which has characteristic features both in clinical signs and on microscopy. It may be acute, subacute or chronic.

The *acute* form is red and swollen with papules, vesicles, exudation, serous crusting, and scaling.

The *chronic* form is red, scaly, thickened, dry and sometimes fissured.

The *subacute* form is intermediate between acute and chronic.

No classification of dermatitis/eczema is entirely satisfactory but there is some advantage to consider three categories: those of more or less **'known' cause**; well-defined morphological and clinical patterns of **unknown cause**; and those which are **unclassified** pending further elucidation by the natural history of the condition or by investigation.

'KNOWN' CAUSES

Contact dermatitis, irritant, (22–26) Results from excessive exposure to skin irritants, e.g. detergents, soaps, alkalis, solvents.

Contact dermatitis, allergic, (27–41) The individual is specifically sensitized to a particular low molecular weight chemical, e.g. nickel, dichromate, rubber chemicals, organic dyes, topically applied antibiotics and other medicaments, and a wide range of chemicals used in industrial and domestic life. Positive diagnosis is by patch test (**38–41**).

Gravitational (stasis, varicose), (42–43) Affects the lower legs as a sequel to increased venous pressure, e.g. from incompetent perforating and varicose veins or deep vein thrombosis. It is often complicated by allergic contact dermatitis to a medicament (**35**), by ulceration (**372**), and by spread to other areas ('secondary spread'), (**69**).

Associated with infection & infestation (44) As a complication of bacterial and fungal infections and especially parasitic infestations, e.g. scabies (**169**) and pediculosis (**44**).

Light-induced (45) On the face, backs of hands, and other exposed areas with relation to sun exposure. Not common but may follow drug ingestion (e.g. phenothazine derivatives, tetracyclines, sulphonamides and sulphonyl-urea hypoglycaemic agents) or topical application of photosensitizing chemicals.

Malabsorption & nutritional (46) Rare.   **Drug** Rare.

UNKNOWN CAUSES

Atopic (47–49) Part of the eczema, asthma, hay fever syndrome. The commonest form of infantile eczema. Affects face, neck and distal flexures, i.e. elbow, wrist and knee flexures.

Seborrhoeic (50–56) Manifested by dandruff, itchy scalp, blepharitis, red scaly patches in naso-labial folds and on ears and neck. Patches on presternal area and interscapular region are common. It is sometimes most marked in the major folds, i.e. the groins and axillae.

Lichen simplex (neurodermatitis), (57–60) Thickened pigmented patches at sites easily accessible to scratching. Worse at times of stress. Common sites, nape in women, just below back of elbow, at side of knee or ankle.

Discoid (nummular), (61–63) Assumes a scattered symmetrical coin-shaped pattern.

Palm & sole, *acute* **(64–66)** Recurrent symmetrical itchy blisters on palms and soles ('pompholyx'). Secondary infection is common. *Chronic* **(67)** Symmetrical, dry, hyperkeratotic, thickened, fissured palms and soles.

'Secondary spread' (68, 69) A patch of eczema anywhere may be complicated by a symmetrical widespread dermatitis which may be discoid or confluent. It often accompanies gravitational eczema and acute palm and sole eczema.

Erythrodermic eczema (70) Generalised dermatitis/eczema with no normal skin areas remaining, which is not generalised psoriasis, reticulosis or other individual dermatosis.

UNCLASSIFIED (71, 72)

Many eczematous eruptions do not fit conveniently into either the unknown or known categories. Their classification must be regarded as pending until investigation is complete.

22 *Irritant contact dermatitis, hand* This shows typical changes of dermatitis : redness, scaling, weeping, vesiculation, hyperkeratosis and fissuring. This pattern is produced by contact with irritants such as strong detergents, soaps, alkalis and solvents. A similar reaction tends to occur under wedding rings. It is *not* an allergic reaction.

23 *Irritant contact dermatitis, lip licking* This child readily demonstrated her technique of lip licking which has produced the lesions, a marginated perioral zone of dry scaly inflammation. It is not uncommon in children but parents will not always accept that lip licking is the cause.

24 *Irritant contact dermatitis, chest* The patient washed her bra using strong bleach and rinsing was incomplete.

22

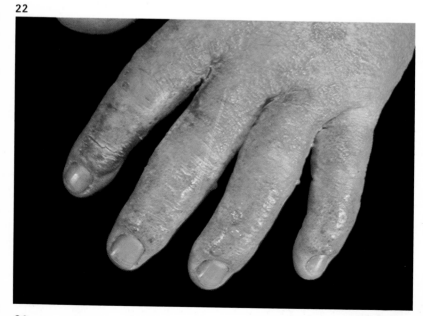

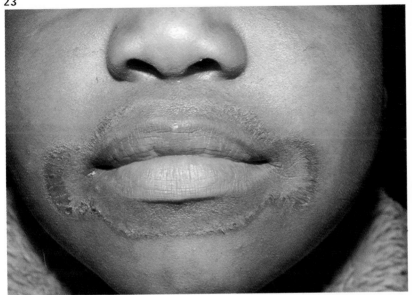

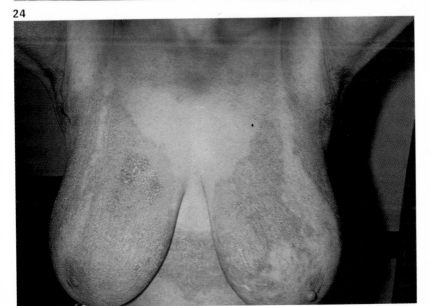

25 *Eczema, irritant contact ('eczéma craquelé') of shin* Over-enthusiastic washing leads to drying and cracking of the stratum corneum. Not infrequently seen in hospital wards, the shins are usually the first to be affected. Avoidance of soap and application of a simple ointment lead to rapid cure.

26 *Eczema, irritant contact ('eczéma craquelé') of shin, close-up* Linear cracking of the stratum corneum produces a mild inflammation.

27 *Allergic contact dermatitis, hair dye* The margins of the scalp are usually most affected. The allergen is paraphenylenediamine (or related chemical), a constituent of many dark dyes. The patient may have used the preparation without ill effects for months or years before sensitization occurs, but once it does each application will lead to dermatitis within 24 – 48 hours.

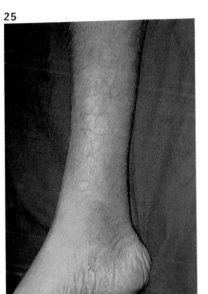

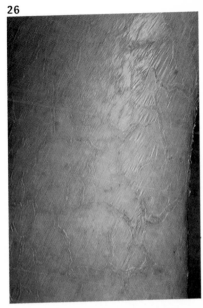

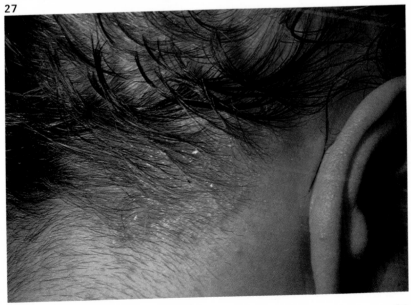

28 *Allergic contact dermatitis, nickel* Patients sensitive to nickel will produce lesions under white metal jewellery or fastenings, e.g. earrings, necklace and bra clips, watch bands and zips. A watch band clasp was responsible in the patient shown. Patch test positive to 5% nickel sulphate solution.

29 *Allergic contact dermatitis, adhesive plaster* The patient was sensitive to colophony resin in adhesive plaster. Blistering is prominent in this case. Patients should be asked about previous adhesive plaster reactions before it is applied. Patch test positive to 20% colophony in soft paraffin.

30 *Allergic contact dermatitis, perfume* Sensitization can occur to one of the essential oils or a 'fixative' (e.g. balsam of Peru) in the perfume.

28

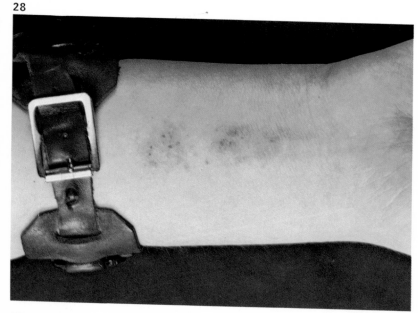

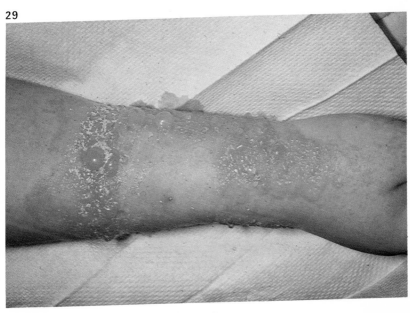

29

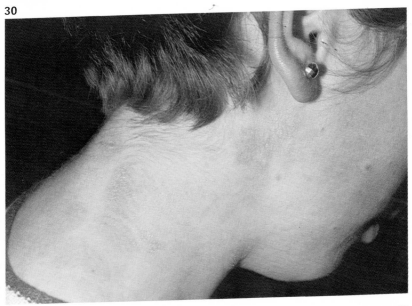

30

31 *Allergic contact dermatitis, nail varnish* The fingers are not affected due to care of application of the varnish but small quantities rub off on the eyelids, face, neck or other areas when they are touched with the fingernails and dermatitis results. Patch test positive. The allergen is an aryl sulphonamide formaldehyde resin.

32 *Allergic contact dermatitis, shoes* The patient did not realize she was sensitive to rubber chemicals in the soles of her shoes. The chemicals (usually mercaptobenzothiazole or tetramethylthiuramdisulphide) are absorbed through to the foot. The pressure points of the sole are the worst affected, and the proximal parts of the toes and the toe-webs are clear. This condition is often misdiagnosed as fungal infection. The treatment is to wear rubber-free footwear. Patch test positive to 1% chemical. The above chemicals are often present in garments containing rubber or rubber substitutes and may give rise to dermatitis at sites of contact.

31

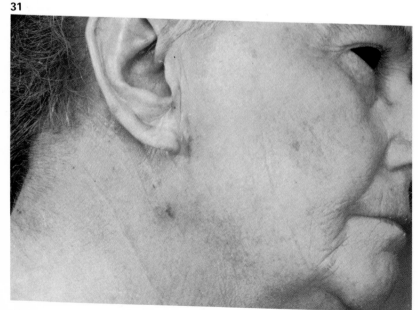

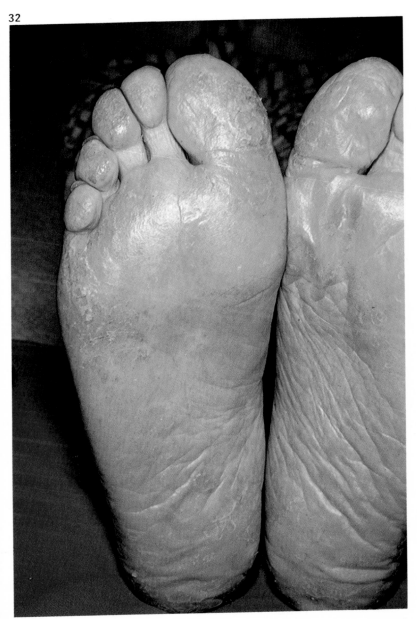

33 *Allergic contact dermatitis, face*   The patient became sensitive to benzylperoxide in a therapeutic face cream. Facial eczema is often very oedematous, especially on the eyelids, and is often misdiagnosed as erysipelas (**86**). Dermatitis is pruritic, an important diagnostic symptom. The white appearance is due to calamine lotion which is not the most cosmetic of treatments for the face.

34 *Allergic contact dermatitis, chrysanthemum*   In addition to lesions on the upper limbs, as shown here, an acute dermatitis of the face may be produced. Examples of plants which can cause allergic contact dermatitis are primula, chrysanthemum, tulip and garlic. In the United States the commonest plant dermatitis is the result of Rhus (poison ivy, poison oak) sensitivity where it presents as streaks and patches of dermatitis, often with blisters.

35 *Allergic contact dermatitis to medicated tulle*   The patient has mild gravitational ulceration. The tulle dressing contained soframycin to which she had become sensitive. Soframycin often cross-reacts with neomycin, which is a fairly common sensitizer.

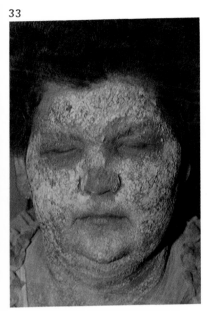

33

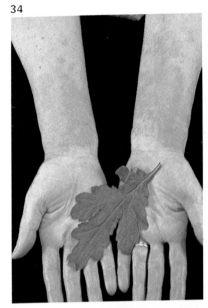

34

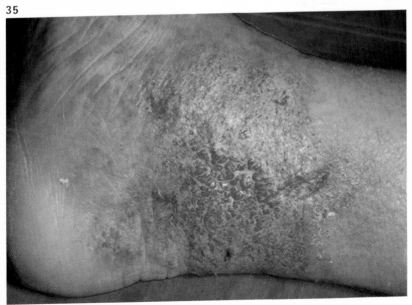

35

36 *Berloque dermatitis, neck and chest* This lesion is caused by perfume containing a *psoralen*, i.e. a chemical which renders the skin sensitive to light at the site of application. The result is inflammation at the site with subsequent post-inflammatory hyperpigmentation. The streaky pattern is typical. The psoralen in perfume is usually bergamot oil.

37 *Tattoo, reaction to red pigment* The patient had an allergic reaction to mercury in the cinnebar pigment.

38 *Patch testing, preparation* To confirm the diagnosis of allergic contact dermatitis, patch testing with appropriate concentrations of a series of common sensitizers is carried out. The chemicals are dissolved in water or in soft paraffin ointment and are applied in sequence to patch test dressings as shown. In addition to the group of chemicals used for all such patients other sensitizers can be tested as suggested by the patient's history, occupation or hobbies. It is most important that the correct concentration of the test substance is used for patch testing (information on this is to be found in dermatological text books and monographs). Some known sensitizers are irritant in high concentration and false-positive reactions can occur.

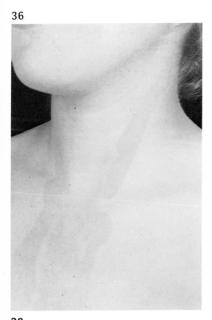

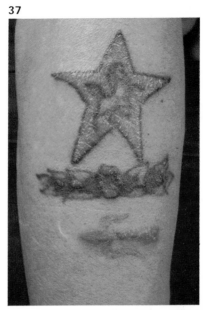

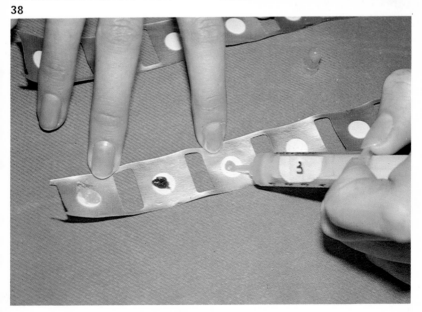

39 & 40 *Patch testing, application* Patch test dressings treated with the desired sequence of chemicals are placed in position on the back (or other convenient part of the skin surface) and are occluded with waterproof adhesive plaster. If the patient is known to be sensitive to the usual adhesive plaster, plastic or paper adhesive tape is used. The tests are left undisturbed for 48 – 72 hours.

41 *Patch testing, results* At the end of 48 – 72 hours the test dressings are discarded and test sites are inspected for inflammation. Positive tests will be pruritic and show erythema and oedema with variable degrees of vesiculation and exudation. A positive patch test indicates allergic sensitivity to the chemical applied. Positive results are recorded and correlated with the patient's eruption and history to determine their exact relevance to the dermatitis under investigation. Shown here are positive patch test reactions to two concentrations of dinitrochloro-benzene (DNCB), a potent sensitizer, with a negative control patch (C).

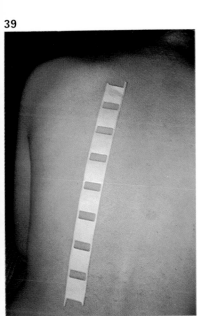

39

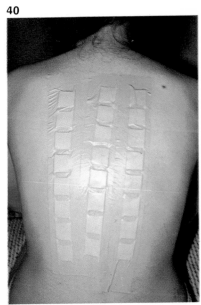

40

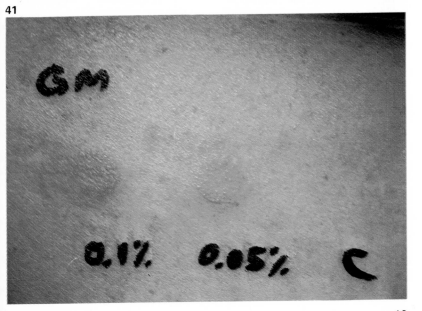

41

42 *Dermatitis, gravitational (stasis, varicose), ankle* This very common form of eczema is usually associated with varicose or incompetent perforating veins of the leg. It is often complicated by oedema, infection, ulceration, allergic contact sensitization to topical medicaments and secondary spread of eczema to the face and other area. The common allergens are lanolin, antibiotics, antibacterial agents and preservatives.

43 *Dermatitis, gravitational (stasis, varicose), acute-on-chronic* Sudden exacerbation of chronic gravitational dermatitis suggests infection or allergic contact sensitization to a medicament.

42

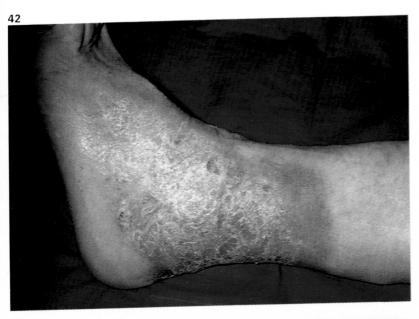

43

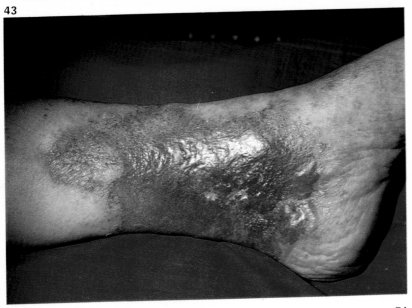

44 *Dermatitis/eczema, associated with infestation* The patient had widespread excoriated chronic eczema. Pediculosis corporis was confirmed by finding lice and eggs in the seams of his clothing (**173**). Scabies may also produce widespread eczema (**169**).

45 *Dermatitis/eczema, light-induced, face* The patient developed an eczematous eruption in sunlight-exposed areas (i.e. the face and backs of the hands). This distribution, where the covered areas are spared, should always raise the suspicion of light sensitivity (see section on light-induced dermatoses).

46 *Eczema due to malabsorption* The patient had patchy eczema and hyperpigmentation associated with steatorrhoea. Lesions show no specific features and the association with malabsorption is not common. The eruption cleared after the patient started a gluten-free diet.

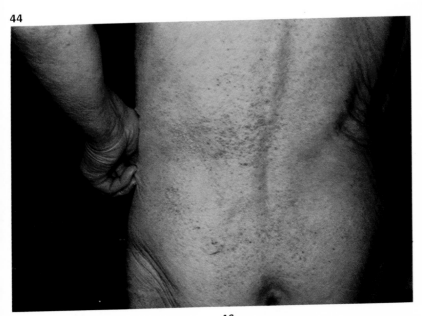

44

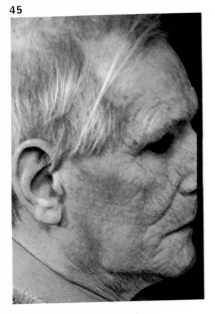

45

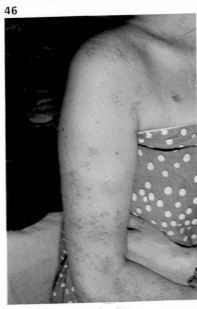

46

53

47 & 48 *Atopic dermatitis, elbow, wrist and knee flexures* This type of dermatitis is often associated with a personal and/or family history of asthma and hay fever. Common in infants and children it tends to settle in the distal flexures (wrist and ankle flexures, elbow and knee flexures) during early childhood. It is the commonest type of so-called 'Infantile eczema'. Lesions are also present on the face and neck. They are very pruritic and when scratched become excoriated and lichenified. The whole skin is usually very dry (atopic xerosis). Atopic dermatitis usually clears by puberty, but may persist for several decades. In dark-skinned patients (**47**) chronic eczema shows inflammatory hyper-pigmentation.

47

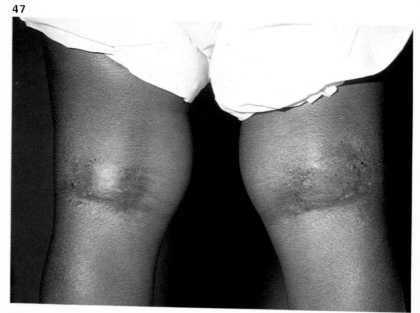

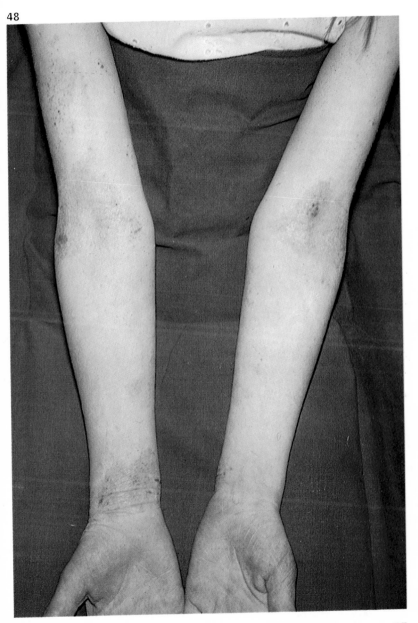

49 *Atopic dermatitis, perioral* The area around the mouth is commonly involved. The vermillion of the lips is dry and scaly. The area adjacent to the centre of the upper lip is often the last to clear. Sometimes in this disorder the whole face is of a uniform pale pink colour with dryness and fine scaling.

50 & 51 *'Seborrhoeic' dermatitis, face, axillae and groins* The term 'seborrhoeic' is anachronistic and not related to aetiology. It is usually used for an eczematous pattern of unknown cause appearing in the axillae and groins, on the scalp, face, neck and ears, and in presternal and interscapular regions. Secondary bacterial infection may occur.

49

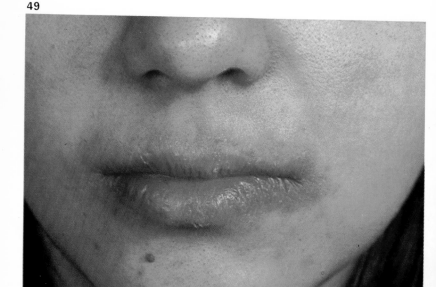

50

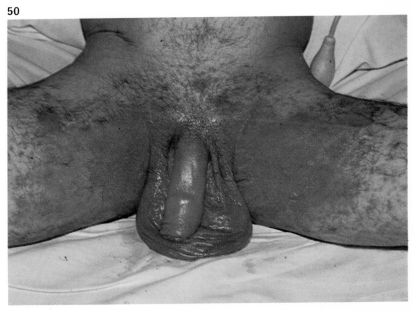

51

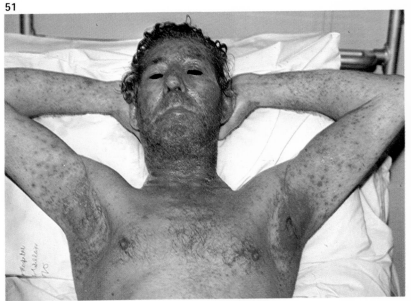

52 *'Seborrhoeic' dermatitis, infantile* The 'napkin (diaper) eruption' is common in infants. It is not usually related to atopic dermatitis and clears within a few weeks with appropriate treatment. It is sometimes called 'napkin psoriasis' but its connection with common psoriasis is uncertain. There are some who regard it as due to candida infection or milk allergy, but conclusive evidence is lacking.

53 *'Seborrhoeic' dermatitis, infantile* More severe napkin (diaper) eruption in a child of Caribbean origin.

54 *Ammoniacal dermatitis, infantile* This napkin (diaper) eruption has become ulcerative due to very poor hygiene. If wet napkins are left in position urine decomposition liberates ammonia which is a skin irritant.

52

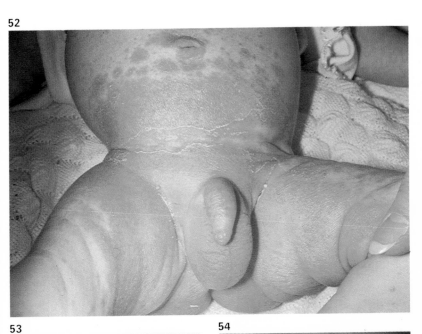

53

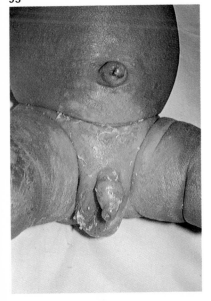

54

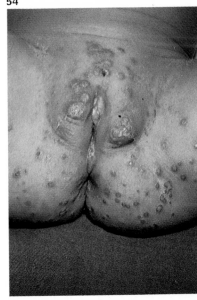

55 *'Seborrhoeic' dermatitis, infantile, scalp and forehead lesions*
Thick greasy scales in the scalp ('cradle cap') and red scaly patches on
the head and neck are often seen in association with napkin (diaper)
eruption.

56 *'Seborrhoeic' dermatitis 'seborrhoeide'* Adults with dandruff
sometimes develop symmetrical brownish scaly patches on the neck and
shoulders. Treating the scalp usually clears the rash.

57 *Lichen simplex ('localised neurodermatitis'), nape of neck*
Tense individuals who scratch a particular area of skin when under stress
often develop a single patch of lichenified eczema. The nape pattern is
virtually seen only in women. It is a thickened plaque with exaggerated
skin markings thrown up in relief.

58 *Lichen simplex, scrotum* A fissured, thickened (lichenified)
eczema is shown. This is sometimes misdiagnosed as a fungal infection.
Mycological examination of skin scrapings is necessary.

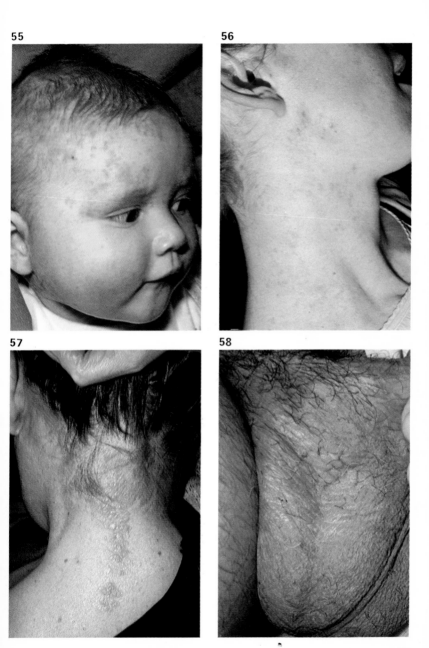

59 *Lichen simplex ('localised neurodermatitis'), lateral shin*
The patient was a telephonist who scratched his left leg with his left
hand when the switchboard became busy. A differential diagnosis would
be hypertrophic lichen planus (**191**).

60 *Lichen simplex, perianal* This is one type of lesion which causes
pruritus ani and it tends to occur in individuals with an 'obsessional' per-
sonality. Pruritus ani may however be due to other causes ; e.g. discharge
from haemorrhoids, allergic contact dermatitis to constituents of topical
applications or suppositories, anal fissures, and excessive sweating.

59

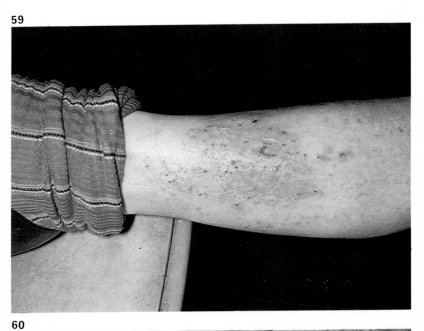

60

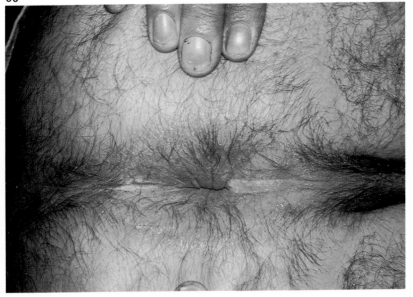

61, 62 & 63 *Discoid eczema (nummular dermatitis), hand, arms and legs* Fairly symmetrical, small round coin-shaped plaques of eczema appear on the limbs, usually on extensor surfaces. Serous crusting is common. Young adults are frequently affected. It is sometimes part of a secondary spread from eczema elsewhere (see **68**) but usually no cause is found. It is not related to atopic eczema.

61

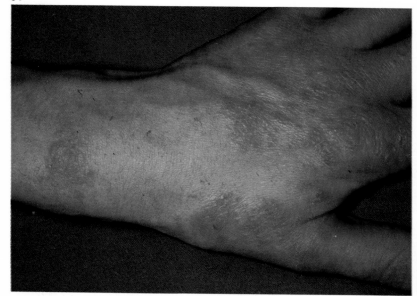

62

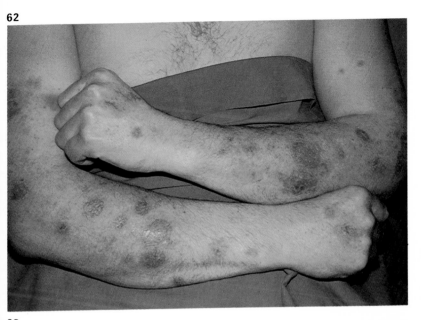

63

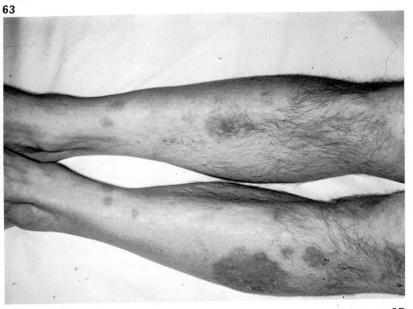

64 *Palm and sole eczema, acute vesicular ('pompholyx'), palms*
A fairly common pattern of eczema which can be recurrent. Usually no
cause is demonstrable but this pattern can be due to trichophytin sensitivity and associated with fungal infection of the feet. Sometimes the
epidermal vesicles resemble sago grains which can only be seen on close
inspection. This patient's blisters were unusually large.

65 *Palm and sole eczema, acute vesicular, soles* The soles were
intensely pruritic. There was no evidence of fungal infection or of allergic
contact eczema.

66 *Palm and sole eczema, acute infected, palm* Secondary infection in acute vesicular eczema of the palms is a common complication. Pus forms in the blisters and the hands are red, swollen and very
painful. Lymphangitis and fever may be present. Staphylococci or strep-
tococci are grown from swabs of the pus.

64

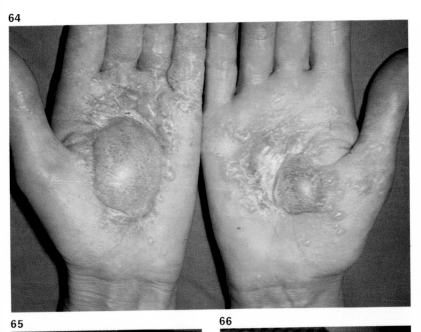

65

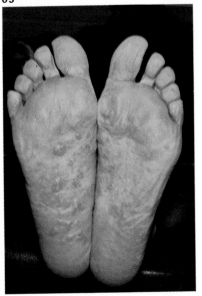

66

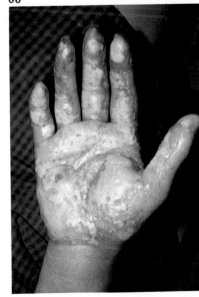

67 *Palm and sole eczema, chronic hyperkeratotic and fissured* This chronic condition may follow on from the acute form or may start in this way. The stratum corneum is thick, dry and brittle so that hand movements result in painful cracks. Avoidance of soap, and a greasy application are indicated.

68 *Dermatitis/eczema, secondary spread* Eczema can spread from the primary site either locally or to give a widespread symmetrical eruption. The patient's primary lesion was on the left wrist and was due to allergic contact dermatitis from a watch strap, which contained nickel.

69 *Dermatitis/eczema, secondary spread, face* The patient presented complaining of the face eruption only. When she undressed it was found that she had an acute-on-chronic gravitational eczema of the left ankle which was the primary lesion. This situation is by no means uncommon and a full examination of the skin is mandatory.

70 *Erythrodermic eczema (exfoliative dermatitis)* Almost any variety of eczema if neglected or treated inappropriately can spread to involve the whole skin surface. Drug eruptions, especially those due to heavy metals, sometimes take this form.

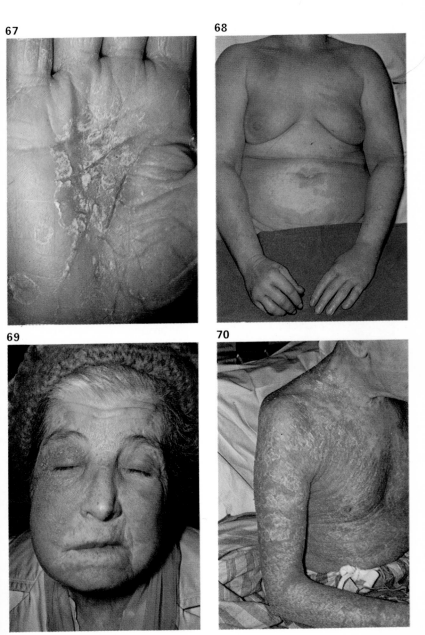

71 *Dermatitis/eczema, unclassified, exfoliative cheilitis* The pattern of eczema in a particular patient may defy classification. Unclassified eczema requires investigation at least to the extent of scraping for fungus and patch testing. No cause was found for this eruption of the lips.

72 *Dermatitis/eczema, unclassified, unilateral nipple* Unilateral eczema of the nipple must be suspected of being Paget's disease of the nipple (intra-duct carcinoma, **331**) until proven otherwise by skin biopsy. In this patient the histology showed only eczema and the condition cleared with treatment.

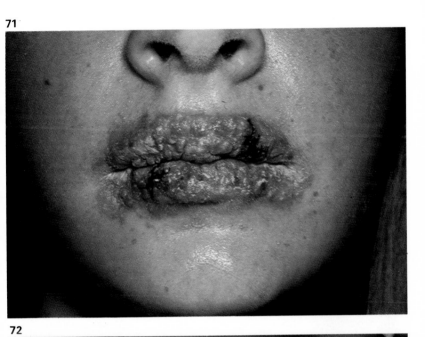

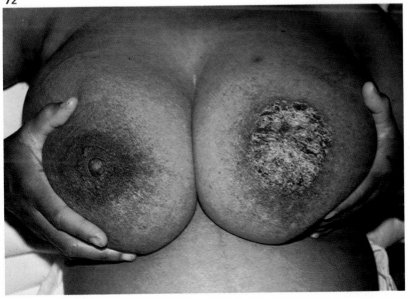

INFECTIONS AND INFESTATIONS

Correct diagnosis of skin infections and infestations is of great importance since curative therapy by specific topical or systemic medicaments is usually readily available, and they may be made worse by corticosteroids.

Bacterial infections
folliculitis **73**
sycosis barbae **74**
furuncle **75, 76**
stye **77**
impetigo contagiosa **78–82**
ecthyma **83**
lymphangitis & cellulitis **84**
erysipelas **85, 86**
septicaemia **87**
dental sinus **88**
syphilis **89–99**
tuberculosis **100–104**
leprosy **105–108**
erythrasma **137,138**

Protozoal infection
leishmaniasis **109**

Fungal infections
tinea capitis **110, 111**
tinea corporis **112–122**

Yeast infections
candidiasis **123–132**
pityriasis versicolor **133–136**

Viral infections
viral warts **139–147**
molluscum contagiosum **148–150**
herpes simplex **151–156**
vaccinia **157–159**
herpes zoster **160–162**

possible viral infections
pityriasis rosea **163–166**
Gianotti-Crosti syndrome **167**

Infestations
scabies **168–172**
pediculosis **173–178**
insect bites **179,180**
creeping eruption **181**

73 *Folliculitis* Hair follicles in adults are liable to become infected with staphylococci. Hairy areas subject to moistness and friction are particularly at risk (e.g. axillae and the back of the neck under the collar). Folliculitis may arise as a complication following the application of a corticosteroid ointment. It starts as a red spot around the follicular orifice, and develops into a superficial pustule.

74 *Folliculitis, sycosis barbae* Shaving in men can spread staphylococcal infection from follicle to follicle. The example shown is relatively mild. Very severe forms, common in the past, are now rarely seen.

73

74

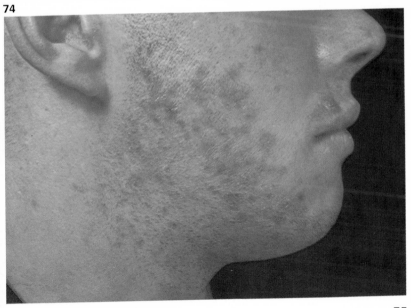

75 *Furuncle (boil)* If the staphylococcal infection of a hair follicle extends throughout its length to be accompanied by intense inflammation and suppuration it is called a furuncle. If several adjacent hair follicles are involved with confluent inflammation it is called a 'carbuncle'. These lesions are very painful.

76 *Furunculosis, axilla* Furunculosis can be a presenting sign of diabetes mellitus and the urine should be tested for sugar.

77 *Stye (hordeolum), lower eyelid* A stye is a boil in an eyelash follicle. Most cases carry pathogenic staphylococci in the anterior nares as well as in the lesion and both require treatment with an antibiotic or antibacterial ointment.

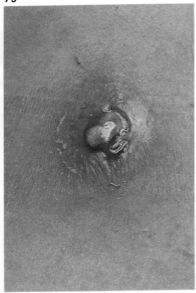

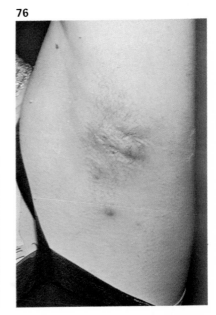

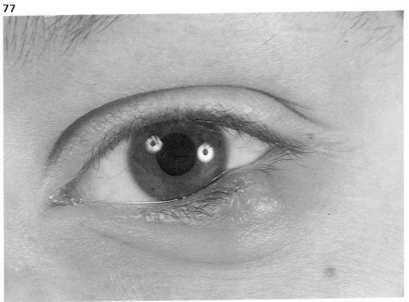

78 *Impetigo contagiosa, face* This is a spreading staphylococcal or streptococcal infection of the epidermis. It is common in children and often spreads from the nostrils which form a reservoir of bacteria for infection. Scratching and personal contact spread the infection, and other members of the family are frequently affected. The condition is common during the summer months. In tropical countries lesions may be widespread and severe and epidemics occur. It clears rapidly with antibiotic ointment. When the predominant organism is the streptococcus, impetigo can be followed by acute glomerulonephritis.

79 *Impetigo contagiosa, circinate lesions, chin*

78

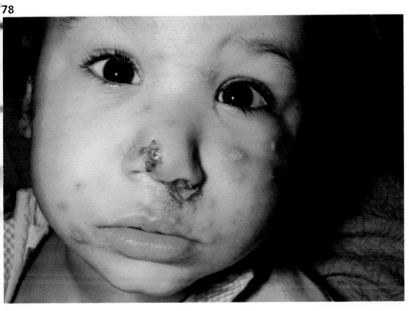

79

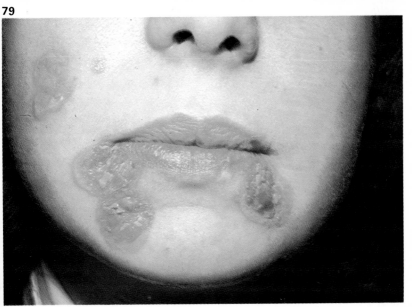

80 *Impetigo contagiosa, face* The superficial nature of the infection and characteristic honey-coloured serous crusting are apparent. Eczema and herpes simplex lesions can become infected and 'impetiginized'.

81 *Impetigo contagiosa* If the infection is of low-grade severity thick serous crusts may form, as on this girl's face.

82 *Bullous impetigo contagiosa, trunk* If the infection spreads rapidly in a young child the stratum corneum is raised to become the roof of a superficial blister, and it ruptures to form an erosion. Blisters and erosions are seen here on the trunk of a child.

83 *Ecthyma* Bacterial infections can produce small, deep, crusted ulcers which eventually heal with scarring. This occurs particularly in the malnourished.

80

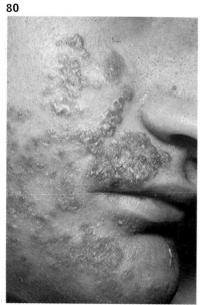

81

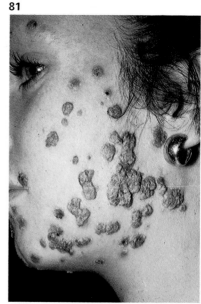

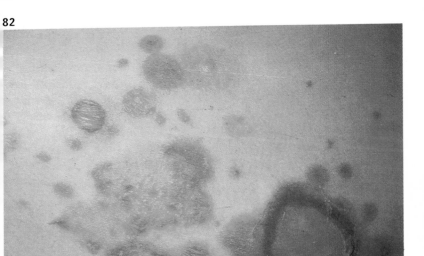

82

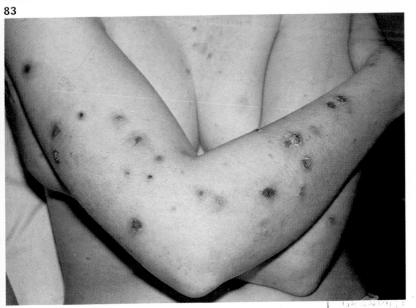

83

84 *Lymphangitis and cellulitis* Tender red streaks up the arm or leg are due to streptococcal infection in lymphatic vessels draining an infected extremity. Common causes are infected eczema of the hands and feet and fungal infection of the toe-webs with fissuring. Enlarged tender lymph nodes in the axillae or groin may be found and high fever with rigors can be associated features. A differential diagnosis is thrombophlebitis.

85 *Erysipelas, leg* The leg is the most common site for this infection. Purpura is common in inflammatory lesions of the legs, whatever the cause.

86 *Erysipelas, face* An acute streptococcal infection with tender erythema and oedema. Recurrent episodes can be associated with increasing lymphoedema.

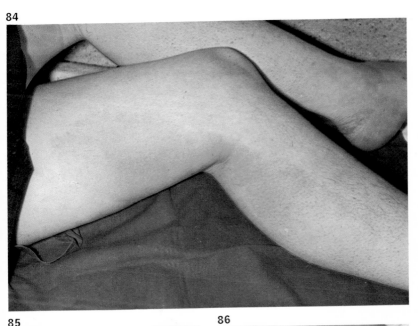

84

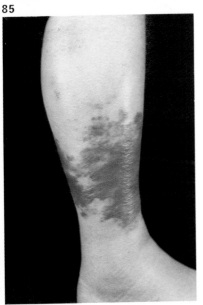

85

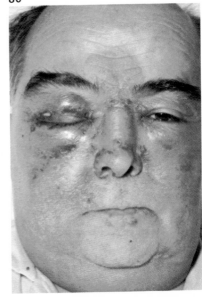

86

87 *Septicaemia* The patient developed extremely tender skin lesions with fever and a positive blood culture following hysterectomy. Individual lesions resemble erythema multiforme (see **349**), but they differ in that they are larger, very tender and irregularly distributed.

88 *Dental sinus* A dental apical abscess can open on the skin anywhere on the face and jaw area to produce a chronic granulating sinus. A typical lesion is shown. Extraction of the infected tooth is curative.

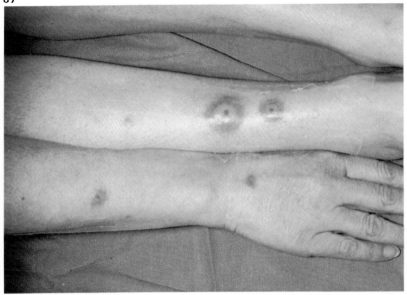

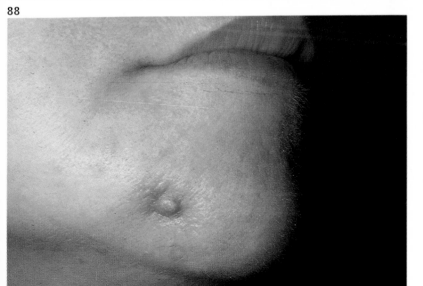

89 *Syphilis, secondary, 'roseola syphilide'* There is a symmetrical profuse eruption of subtle pink macules and barely raised papules at all stages of development. Examination in daylight is usually necessary to see this eruption, it can be completely missed in artificial light. The papular element is best seen here on the patient's left side where the light strikes it obliquely. Patients with secondary syphilis usually feel generally unwell; this can be a helpful diagnostic point in association with other evidence. Pruritus is minimal or absent.

90 *Syphilis, secondary* This is at a later stage of development than in **89**. Scattered papules are seen. The patient felt unwell and had a generalised lymphadenopathy.

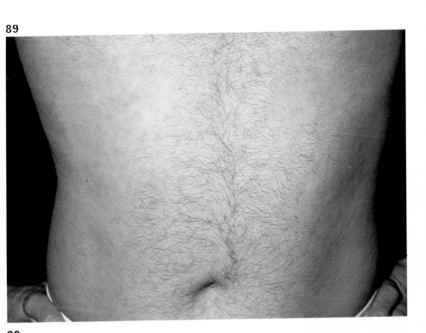

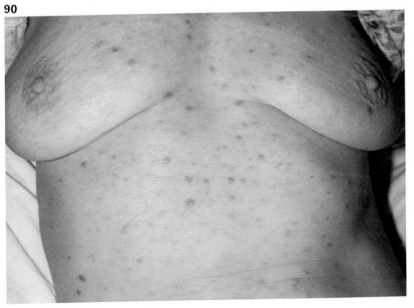

91 *Syphilis, secondary, trunk* This florid eruption resembled a 'toxic' erythema (see **344**).

92 *Syphilis, secondary* Individual papules may resemble psoriasis. The whole skin surface and mucous membranes must be examined. Serology is always strongly positive in secondary lues.

93 *Secondary syphilis, palms* Smooth-topped or scaly symmetrical, brownish papules on the palms and soles are a feature of late secondary syphilis. Patchy loss of scalp hair may also be found.

91

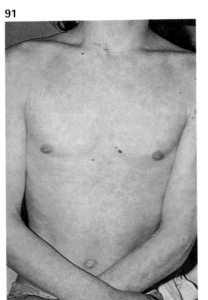

92

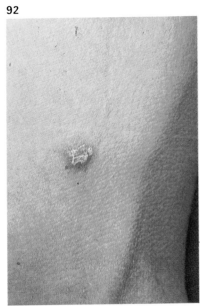

93

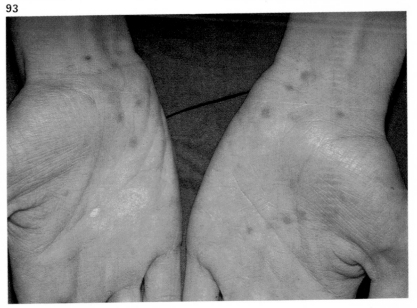

94 *Secondary syphilis, soles*   These papules are similar to those on the palms.

95 *Secondary syphilis, mucous patches, mouth*   Two mucous patches are present to the left of the tip of the tongue. They are super-ficial erosions covered by a thin white slough. The whitish membrane is easily scraped off. They can arise on any part of the tongue or oral mucosa and are usually painless. Treponemes abound in these lesions.

96 *Secondary syphilis, condylomata lata*   Syphilitic raised papules ('warts') occur in the perineum or in any moist intertriginous site. These lesions teem with spirochaetes, they are therefore dark-ground positive and highly contagious. They must be distinguished from viral warts in this area, i.e. condylomata acuminata (**144**).

94

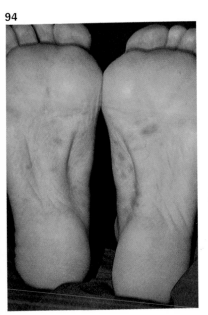

95

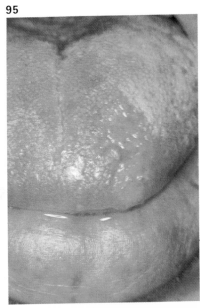

96

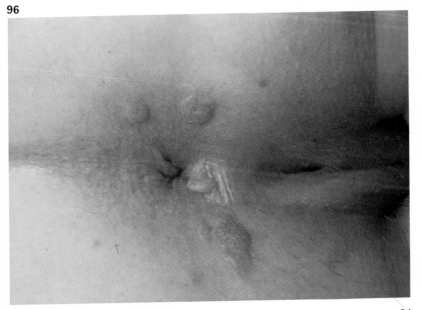

97 *Syphilis, gumma* Note central clearing and extending nodular margin. The lesion was symptomless.

98 *Syphilis, gumma of back* A less florid example than in **97**, but central clearing, peripheral extension and nodulation are still obvious.

99 *Syphilis, ulcerated gumma of calf* The blood Wasserman reaction, or other serological test for syphilis, is an essential investigation in all chronic leg ulcers.

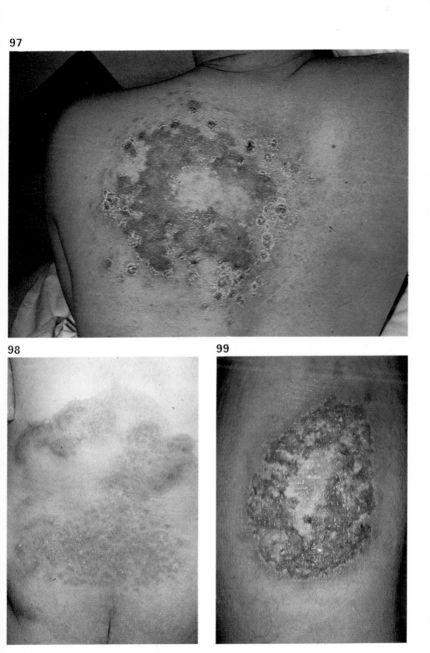

100 *Lupus vulgaris, cheek* Cutaneous tuberculosis in a patient with a strongly positive tuberculin test. The lesion had been growing un-treated for nearly 20 years. It was symptomless. It consisted of clusters of raised brownish-red papules. Atrophy and scarring also occur, particularly after treatment.

101 *Lupus vulgaris, diascopy* Individual granulomatous tubercles are shown up by pressing a microscope slide or transparent spatula over the lesion. The procedure squeezes out the blood from the lesion and small translucent brownish papules are seen. They are sometimes called 'apple jelly' nodules.

100

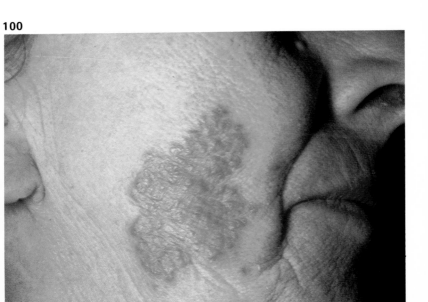

101

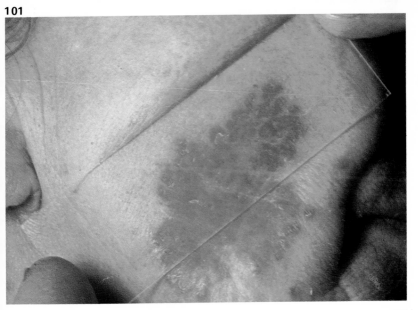

102 *Lupus vulgaris* Lesions producing severe tissue destruction were not uncommon before the advent of antituberculous therapy. Squamous carcinoma can develop on the scarred areas.

103 *Tuberculosis, verrucous* Lesions may be extremely hyperkeratotic and with a warty surface.

104 *Tuberculide, papulonecrotic* Symmetrical, breaking-down granulomatous papules appear on the limbs. The tubercle bacillus is not found in these lesions. The tuberculin reaction is always strongly positive.

102

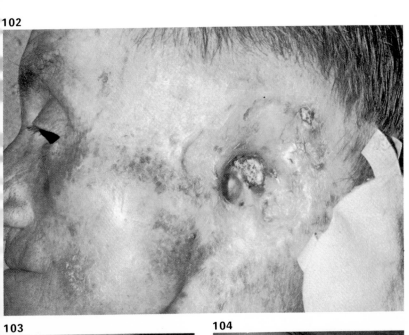

103

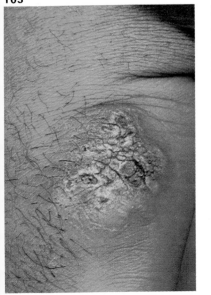

104

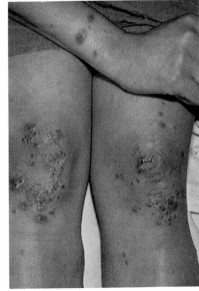

105 *Leprosy, tuberculoid* The patient had a single hypopigmented, analgesic, annular lesion with an indurated edge. Leprosy bacilli are very scanty in these lesions. The lepromin skin test was strongly positive.

106 *Leprosy, lepromatous* Nodular granulomatous lesions on the face are seen. These lesions, which may be scattered over the whole skin surface, contain large numbers of *Mycobacterium leprae*. They can be demonstrated by appropriate staining of a biopsy or of scrapings taken from the sides of an incision extending into the dermis.

107 *Leprosy, borderline* Several annular lesions are present. In borderline and tuberculoid leprosy peripheral nerves are thickened and hard. Peripheral nerve thickening, a physical sign readily elicited, confirms the diagnosis of leprosy.

105

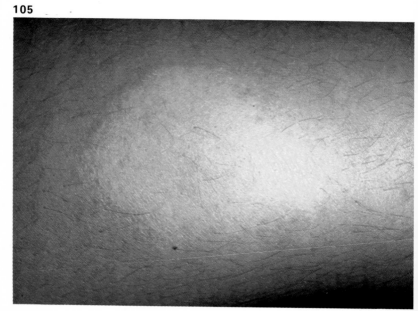

106

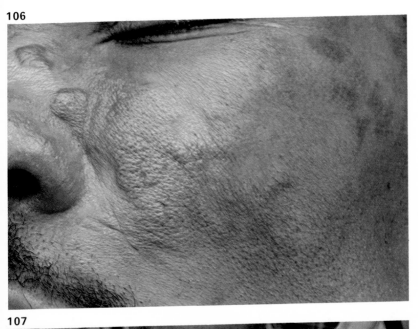

107

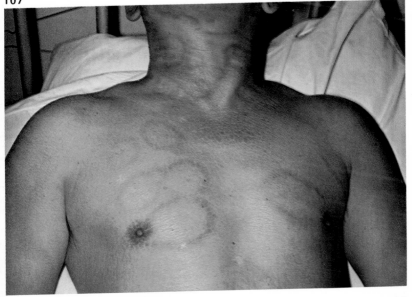

108 *Erythema nodosum leprosum, forearm* The patient has lepromatous leprosy with superimposed erythema nodosum leprosum. These acutely inflamed nodules were extremely tender and the patient was pyrexial.

109 *Cutaneous leishmaniasis ('oriental sore'), cheek* A granuloma caused by the protozoön, *Leishmania tropica,* and transmitted by sandfly bites. Common among inhabitants of the Mediterranean littoral, the Middle East, India and South America, and in those who travel there. The organisms can be stained in deep skin smears and in skin biopsies. The incubation period may be up to two years. If untreated it eventually heals spontaneously to leave a prominent scar. The Leishmanin test is positive.

108

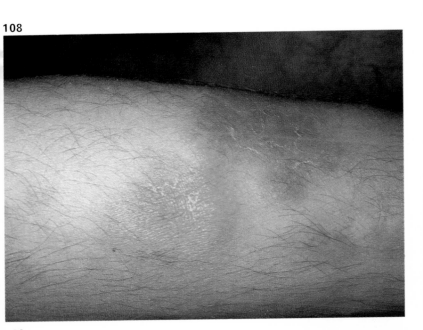

109

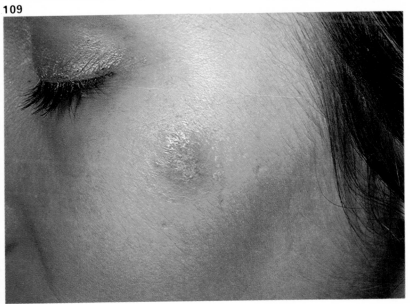

110 & 111 *Tinea capitis (fungal infection), scalp ringworm*

Fungal scalp infections are confined largely to children. The affected hairs are broken off. The scalp surface shows scaling, inflammation and sometimes pustule formation. Most examples due to microsporum species fluoresce green under Wood's light in a darkened room. Affected hairs and scrapings from the area will demonstrate fungus by microscopy and by culture on nutrient agar.

Sometimes very severe inflammation in these patches results in a tender boggy mass ('kerion') ; if this happens the infection is cured but scarring alopecia may be produced (**260**).

An extensive patch in the left parietal region (**111**). It could easily be mistaken for alopecia areata (see **252**) but fungus was found in scrapings.

112 *Tinea pedis (fungal infection), toes* There is scaling in the toe-webs but, in this patient, no obvious inflammation. If untreated, toe-web fungus can spread to produce inflammation of the toes, feet, groins, and more distant sites.

110

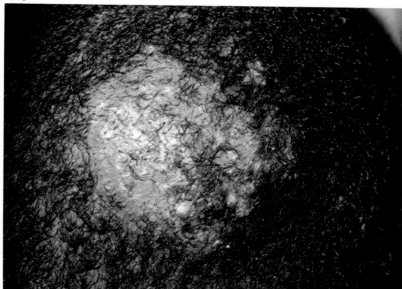

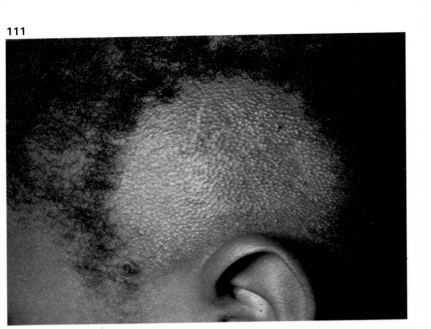

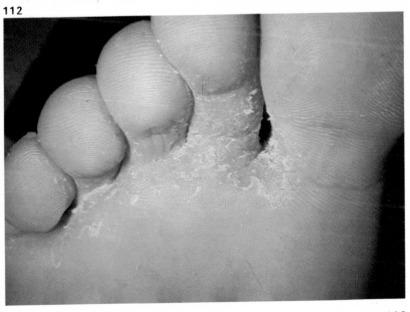

113 *Tinea pedis (fungal infection), toe-web* The moist environment of the toe-webs is a favourite site for maceration and fungal infection. Itching is a prominent symptom.

114 *Tinea pedis (fungal infection), dorsal foot* Spread of inflammation from the toe-webs to adjacent skin on the foot frequently occurs and is a helpful diagnostic sign.

115 *Tinea cruris (fungal infection), groin* The groin is a favoured site for ringworm in men. An itchy scaly lesion with an advancing arcuate edge is found. The toe-webs and finger and toenails should also be examined for infection.

116 *Tinea corporis (fungal infection), dorsal hand* Annular lesions (hence 'ringworm') are found on exposed skin areas.

113

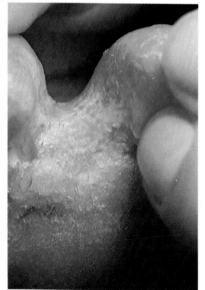

114

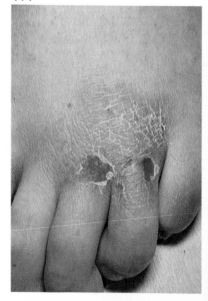

115

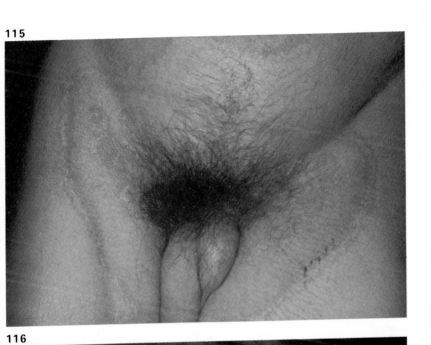

116

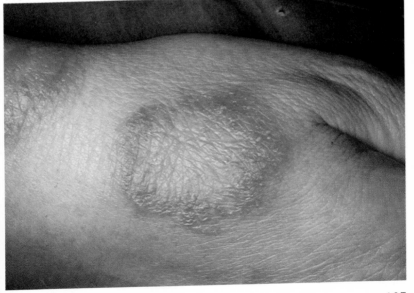

117 *Tinea corporis (fungal infection), thigh, exacerbated by topical steroid* A topical steroid ointment was applied to this lesion. It partially suppressed itching and scaling but did not prevent it extending. Topical corticosteroids are contra-indicated in fungal infections.

118 *Tinea unguium (fungal infection), fingernails* The free edges of the nails are dystrophic, brittle, thickened and separated from the underlying nail plate (onycholysis). To confirm the diagnosis, clippings from affected nails are cultured on Sabouraud's medium (glucose agar). Toenails are more frequently affected than fingernails. The condition is only rarely symmetrical and often only one or two nails are involved.

119 *Tinea corporis (fungal infection), palms* The left palm is slightly scaly. Palmar infection with *Trichophyton rubrum* can be very extensive with minimal physical signs.

117

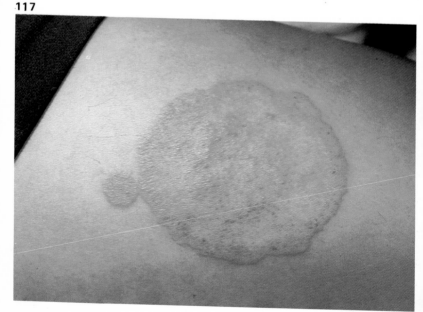

118

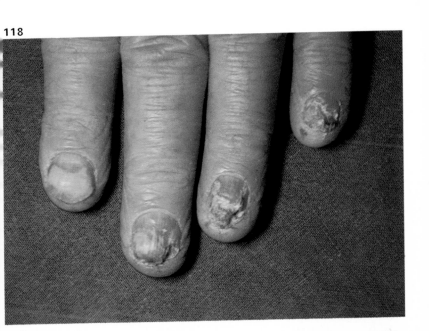

119

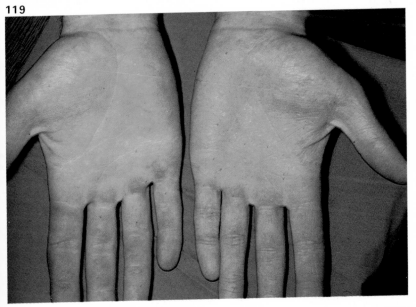

120 *Tinea corporis, scraping for fungus*   The patient has a red scaly eruption on his dorsal wrist. Scales from the edge of the lesion are being gently scraped onto a glass slide using a blunt scalpel. The scales are mounted in 10%–30% potassium hydroxide solution under a cover-slip, and are examined under the low power of the microscope with the sub-stage iris diaphragm almost closed.

121 *Fungus, microscopy of scrapings*   There are long threads of mycelium, some branched, running through the scale. The threads are refractile and their dark edges give them a characteristic appearance of railway lines. Threads which are out of focus are dark but are still distinctive.

122 *Tinea corporis (fungal infection), face*   The eruption is marginated but shows little scaling. It was exacerbated by the application of a corticosteroid ointment.

120

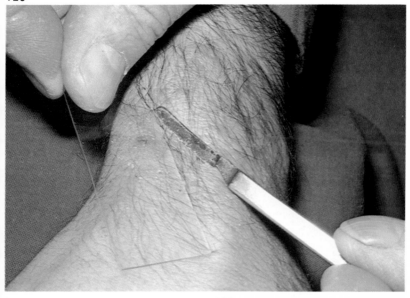

121

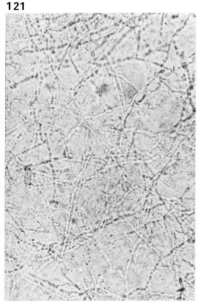

122

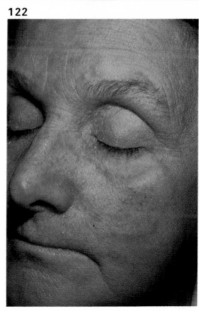

123 *Candida infection, submammary* A common condition beneath pendulous breasts in the elderly. Numerous seborrhoeic warts are also present in this particular patient.

124 *Candidiasis, submammary* Acute candida infections are often pustular. The presence of small pustules scattered beyond the margin of the main lesion is diagnostic.

125 *Angular cheilitis (angular stomatitis)* This common condition is usually due to lack of teeth or poorly fitting dentures producing folds of skin at the corners of the mouth which soon become macerated and infected. More rarely it is the result of a vitamin deficiency. Candida albicans is the usual infective organism.

123

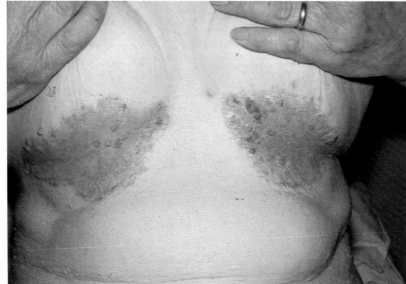

124

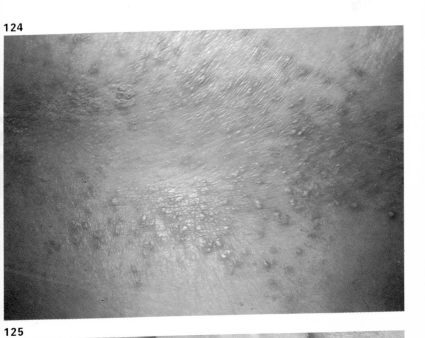

125

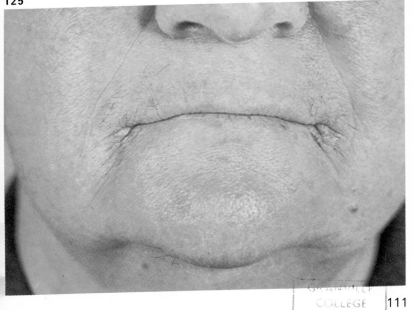

126 *Candida, microscopy* In addition to hyphal threads of candida pseudomycelium there are numerous candida spores present.

127 *Candidiasis, tongue* Buccal candidiasis is common in patients taking systemic antibiotics or cytotoxic agents, or may arise in conjunction with a debilitating illness. Any part of the tongue or oral mucosa can be affected. The white patches are easily scraped off with a spatula to leave a red sore surface.

128 *Candidiasis, groin* The vulval area is itchy, red and oedematous. The infection can be secondary to vaginal candidiasis. It may be a presenting sign of diabetes mellitus and the urine should always be tested for sugar.

129 *Candida infection ('erosio interdigitale')* Finger-web maceration due to wet work and insufficient drying, is the predisposing cause.

126

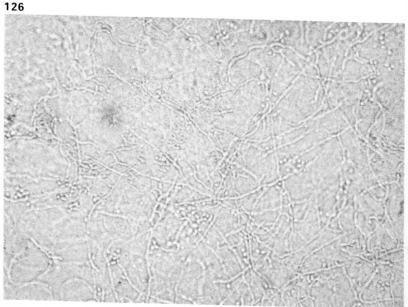

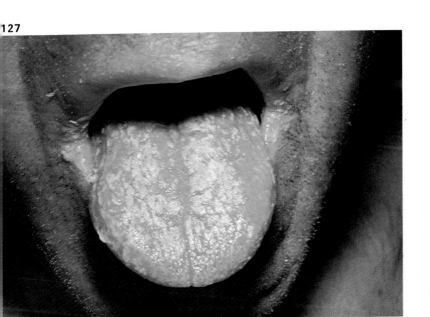

127

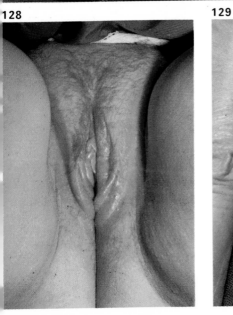

128

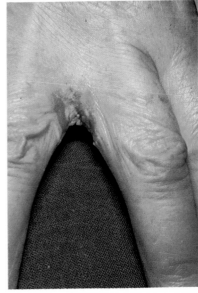

129

130 *Chronic paronychia* The nail fold is damaged and loses its 'cuticle'; water, irritant bacteria and yeasts can then enter the pocket between the nail fold and nail plate. A subacute infection ensues in which *Candida albicans* usually predominates. The result is erythema and oedema (bolstering) of the nail fold with tenderness and often secondary nail dystrophy. General causes are wet manual occupations, poor circulation and over-enthusiastic manicuring. It should *never* be incised surgically. Avoidance of predisposing factors and application of an antibacterial and candidacidal ointment allows the inflammation to resolve and the tissues to return to normal after about three months of treatment.

131 *Chronic paronychia* In this Negro patient the loss of cuticle is evident and the nail plate is dystrophic and hyperpigmented.

132 *Candidiasis, fingernails* Extensive candida infection of the nail plate is rare. Pathological examination of nail clippings is necessary to confirm the infecting organism.

130

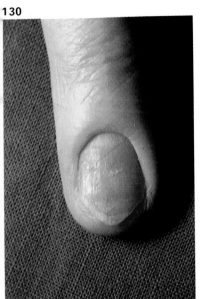

131

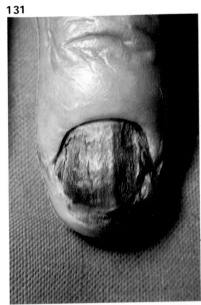

132

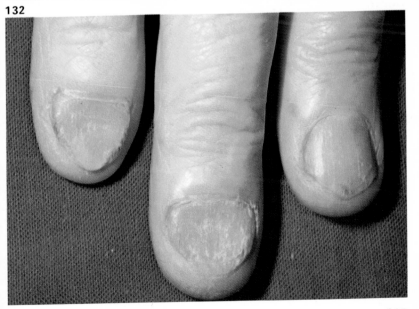

133 & 134 *Pityriasis versicolor, chest* Asymptomatic or itchy macules with a velvety surface of altered pigmentation which scales readily on scraping. Caused by a yeast *Malassezia furfur*. Very common in warm climates. The upper trunk and neck are favoured sites. Untreated it may persist unchanged for many years. In **134** the lesion on the right has been partially scraped to demonstrate the finely scaling surface.

135 *Pityriasis versicolor, shoulder* Dappled hypopigmented or hyperpigmented lesions of the upper trunk are characteristic of this condition. In Negro or dark-skinned subjects lesions are usually darker than surrounding skin due to inflammatory hyperpigmentation. In sun-tanned, fair-skinned subjects lesions are usually lighter than the surrounding skin.

136 *Pityriasis versicolor, microscopy of scales* There are short curved hyphal threads which resemble tangled wool. In addition are seen clusters of spores. This is stained, but the same detail can be readily seen in unstained specimens mounted in 10%–30% KOH solution.

133

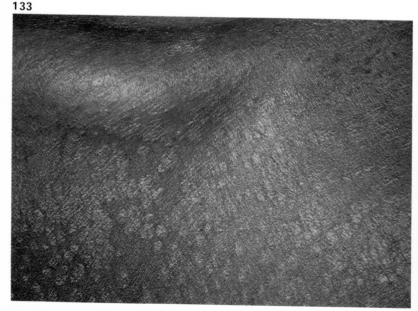

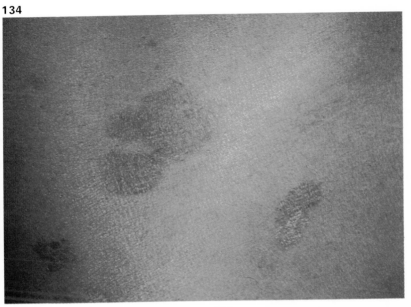

134

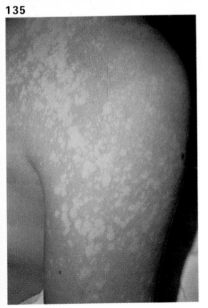

135

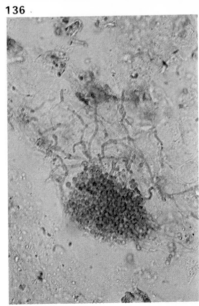

136

137 *Erythrasma, groin* Caused by a bacillus *Corynebacterium minutissimum*, it is found in the groins, axillae and toe-webs, especially in diabetics. Fluoresces coral red under Wood's light.

138 *Erythrasma, axilla* Marginated hyperpigmented lesions are seen.

137

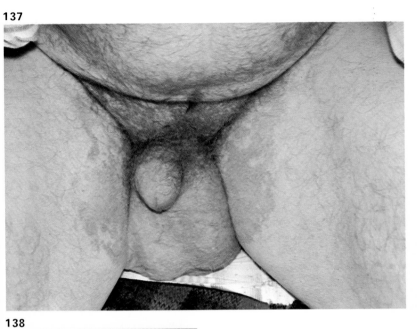

138

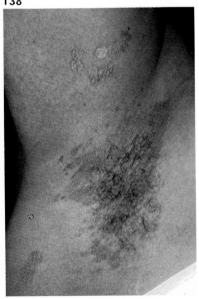

119

139 *Viral warts (Verruca vulgaris), back of hand* Hard well-circumscribed raised rough hyperkeratotic papules.

140 *Viral warts, plantar* These lesions are hyperkeratotic. When a plantar wart is pared down with a scalpel blade soft opalescent wart tissue is revealed.

141 *Plantar viral wart, resolving* The blood vessels in the wart have thrombosed and dark brown spots in the lesion are seen.

142 *Viral wart, Köbner phenomenon, palm* A scratch resulted in a linear wart due to inoculation of virus.

139

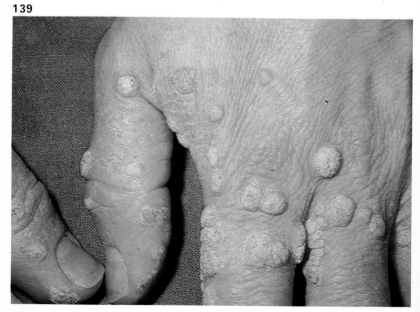

140

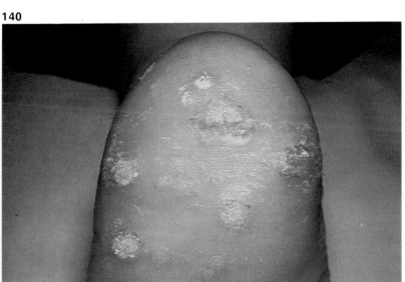

141

142

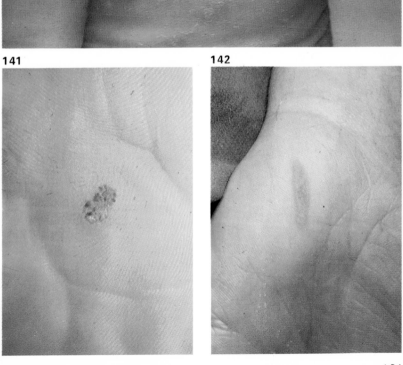

143 *Viral plane warts, group on the back of the hand* Lesions are small, well-demarcated, rather irregular in outline, only slightly elevated and have a matt smooth surface. The forehead and face are other favoured sites for plane warts. They are notoriously resistant to treatment.

144 *Viral warts, perianal (Condylomata acuminata)* There are groups of soft papilliferous tumours. This patient did not delay seeking advice, and at this stage lesions are easily treated by topical cauterising applications. Lesions can usually be differentiated from the condylomata lata of secondary syphilis (**96**).

143

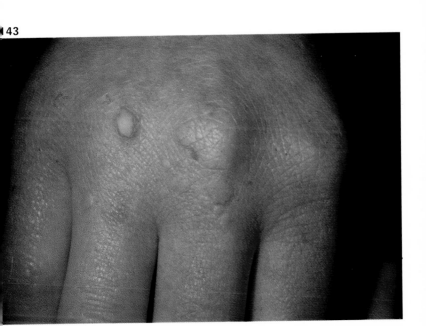

144

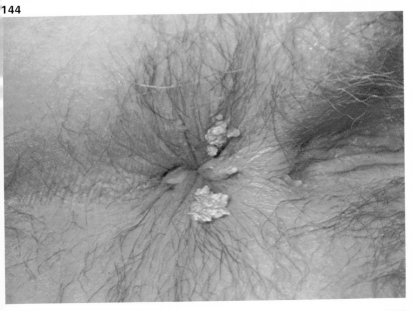

145 *Viral warts, perianal, severe* These large cauliflower-like growths may require surgical treatment under general anaesthetic.

146 *Viral wart, lip* Warts on and around the lips are often secondary to warts on the fingers in children. Smaller, often filiform, lesions are seen in the beard area of adult men who are continually re-inoculated by shaving.

147 *Viral warts, condylomata acuminata, penis* Similar lesions are seen on the vulva.

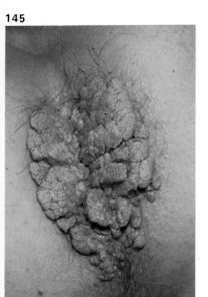

145

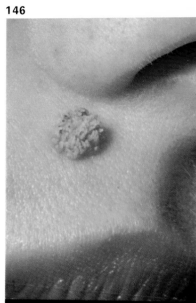

146

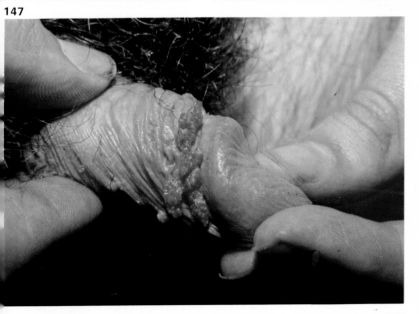

147

148 *Molluscum contagiosum, group on trunk* These are caused by a very large virus and appear as clusters of pearly papules which become umbilicated as they grow. They are commoner in children than in adults. Cheesy contents expressed onto a slide and stained with haematoxylin will show diagnostic 'molluscum bodies' which are infected cytopathic epidermal cells. The Köbner phenomenon may occur.

149 *Molluscum contagiosum, glabella* Lesions around the eyelids are common.

150 *Molluscum contagiosum, forehead* The umbilication of the larger lesion is clearly seen.

148

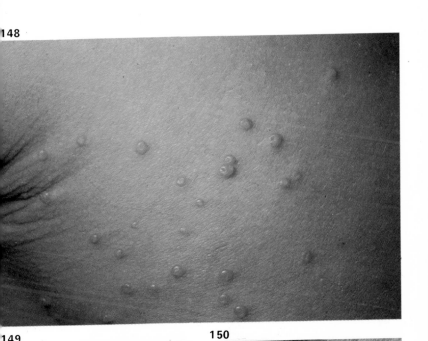

149

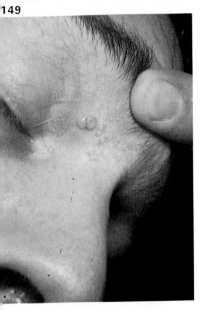

150

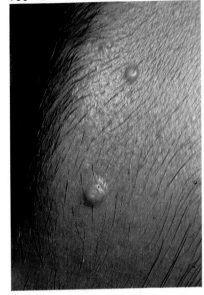

127

151 *Herpes simplex, primary infection* The primary infection in children is often associated with sore gums, buccal ulceration and fever.

152 *Herpes simplex, lips* There are clusters of small vesicles with oedema, pruritus and tenderness. The lips are the most common site for this infection which can be provoked by a febrile illness, by strong sunlight and possibly by psychological factors. The blisters soon rupture to leave serous crusts. Sometimes they become impetiginized.

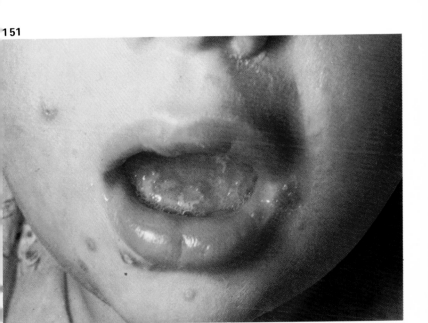

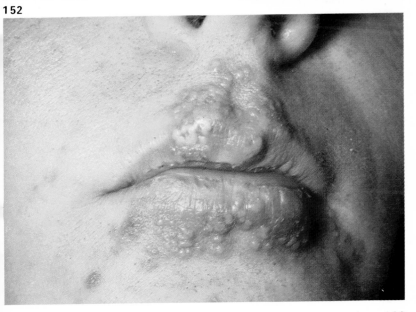

153 *Herpes simplex, cheek* The geographical margin is typical. Any part of the skin surface can be affected by herpes simplex, which may be recurrent at one site.

154 *Herpes simplex, genital, vulva* The superficial red, sharply-marginated ulceration is typical. The condition is intensely painful and may be recurrent. It can complicate pregnancy. In men recurrent lesions may occur on the glans penis or prepuce.

155 *Herpes simplex, buttock* The lesion had been present for several days. In the upper lesion the vesicles have coalesced and become pustular. In the lower lesion the vesicles have ruptured and there is slight serous crusting. A surrounding zone of erythema is commonly seen.

156 *Herpes simplex, eczema herpeticum (Kaposi's varicelliform eruption)* This widespread eruption is a complication of atopic eczema and a few other rarer dermatoses. Due to primary infection with the virus, it can occur even in patients whose atopic eczema is quiescent.

153

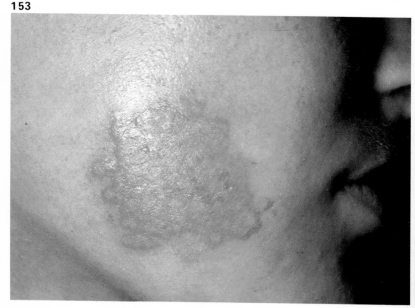

154

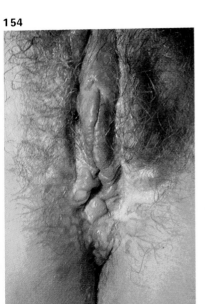

155

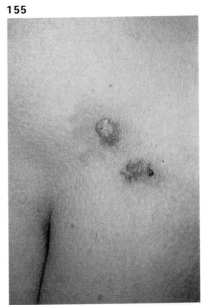

156

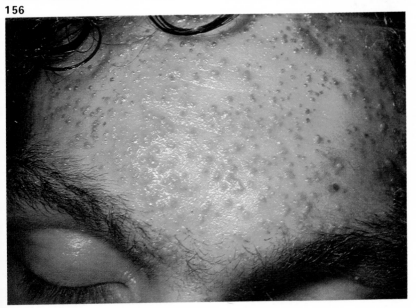

157 *Vaccinia, primary lesion* The vaccinial pustule arises about 10 days after primary vaccination. It dries to leave a scab and eventually a scar. In revaccination a lesion comes within a few days ; it is usually rather small, pruritic, and resolves more quickly.

158 *Vaccinia, accidental, lower eyelid* Vaccinia virus can be implanted into normal skin by the patient, following touching or scratching of the original vaccination site at a time when it is still moist. Characteristic vaccinia pustules are produced. The eyelid is a typical site.

159 *Eczema vaccinatum (Kaposi's varicelliform eruption)* A complication of atopic dermatitis. The patient, usually a child, has recently been either inadvisably vaccinated against smallpox with live vaccinia virus, or has come into contact with an individual with an active vaccinial lesion. Profuse clusters of umbilicated vaccinial vesicles and pustules arise on affected skin.

157

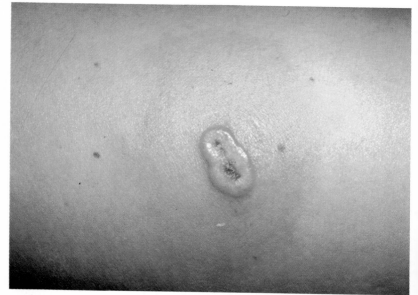

158

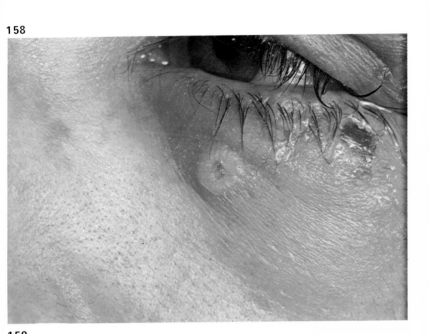

159

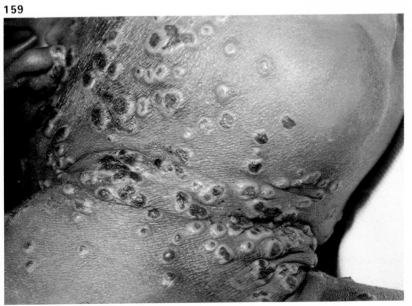

133

160 *Herpes zoster, T7 and T8 nerve roots* There are clusters of small vesicles on a deeply erythematous background with associated oedema, local mild erythema and, in this patient, a widespread 'toxic' erythema. Scattered single vesicles or pustules in other areas are commonly found.

161 *Herpes zoster, ophthalmic and maxillary 5th cranial nerve distribution* A history of pain in the exact distribution of one or more adjacent nerve roots, followed by an eruption of blisters confined to the same anatomical distribution is diagnostic. In this situation severe inflammation of the eye may occur and expert ophthalmological help should be sought at an early stage.

162 *Herpes zoster* The distribution of lesions may be very patchy. In elderly patients lesions may heal with considerable scarring, and post-herpetic neuralgia can cause recurrent severe hyperaesthesia, pain and tenderness at the site for a period of months or years. Severe, ulcerative, haemorrhagic or disseminated herpes zoster is a complication of Hodgkin's disease and other lymphomas.

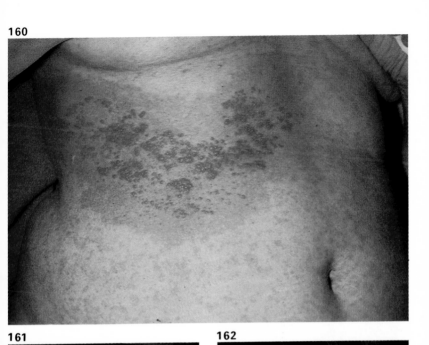

160

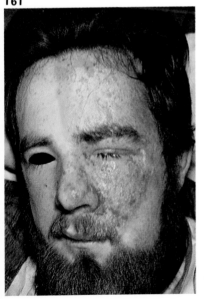

161

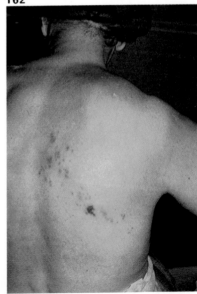

162

163 & 164 *Pityriasis rosea, herald patch, abdomen, trunk* Common in children and young adults especially in spring and autumn months. Is often preceded by a single large lesion, the 'herald patch'. In **163** the herald patch was prominent. Smaller lesions arising subsequently were typical but sparse. In **164** there is a profuse eruption of oval pink macules with marginal scaling with a tendency to be arranged in horizontal lines. Itching is variable and lesions disappear spontaneously in 4 – 6 weeks. A viral aetiology has not been proven.

An important differential diagnosis is secondary syphilis (**90**).

163

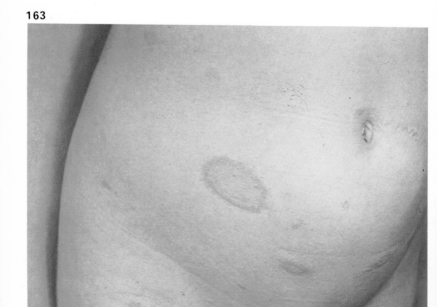

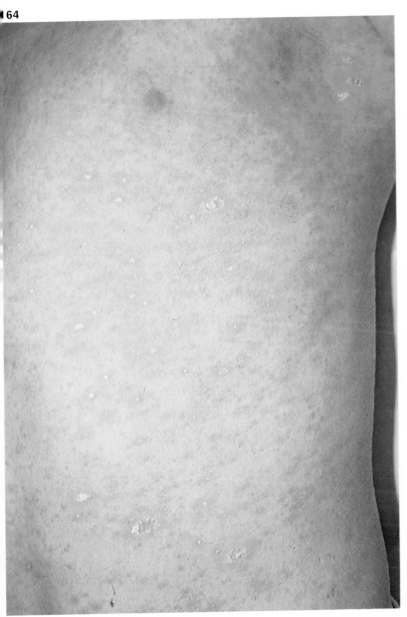

165 *Pityriasis rosea, neck* Sometimes lesions are confined to the neck, groins and upper thighs. There are oval scaly macules in the lines of the skin creases. Some inflammatory hyperpigmentation is also present.

166 *Pityriasis rosea, back* On the back lesions tend to follow the lines of the ribs to give a 'fir tree' appearance. Scaling is very apparent in Negroes, and erythema may be inconspicuous.

167 *Gianotti-Crosti syndrome, forearm* A rare symmetrical eruption of small red papules in infants and young children. It usually starts on the legs, thighs and buttocks and spreads to the arms. Lymph nodes, liver and spleen are sometimes enlarged. It fades spontaneously in 2–8 weeks.

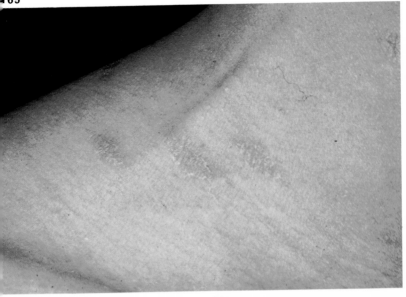

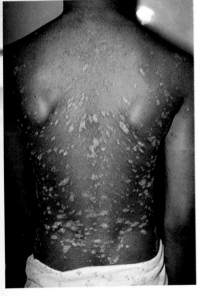

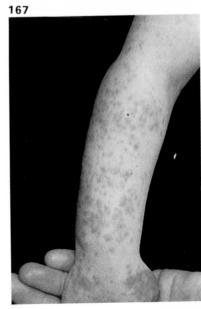

168 *Scabies, burrows on side of finger* The causal mite, *Acarus (Sarcoptes) scabiei var. hominis* is only found in *burrows*. The burrows shown here are unusually prominent. The distribution of lesions gives the clue ; itchy excoriated papules in finger-webs and on fingers, hands, elbows, anterior axillary folds, nipples in women, penis and scrotum in men, buttocks and ankles. The face is always spared except in babies. It must be emphasized that burrows can be very scanty, especially in adults, and prolonged search of all the above areas may be necessary. Burrows are often more easily felt than seen by the examiner.

The diagnosis is confirmed by scraping off an intact papule or burrow onto a drop of 10 – 30% potassium hydroxide solution, mounting it on a slide and searching for the scabies mite and eggs under the lower power of the microscope. The patient's immediate family or sleeping partner is almost certain to be infected, and the history of itching in a contact can be very important diagnostically. If a large family presents for examination it is best to start with the children, since they tend to have more numerous burrows. All members of the family and sleeping partners must receive treatment even if some of them are not apparently infected.

169 *Scabies, eczematised hand lesions* A patchy excoriated fissured eczema of the hands and especially the finger-webs must raise the suspicion of scabies. Usually other members of the family will be itching. If the diagnosis is unsuspected the eczematous reaction may become widespread and severe.

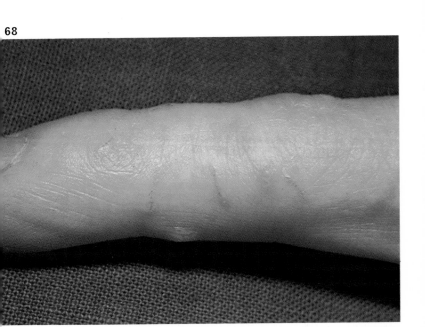

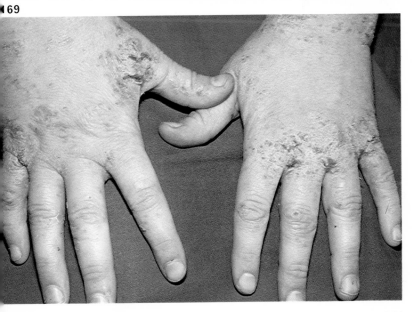

170 Scabies, elbow Burrows and eczematisation are seen.

171 Scabies, penis Papules and burrows on the penis and scrotum are more red and oedematous than those on the hands. They are pathognomonic.

172 Scabies mite and egg The discovery of even a single mite or egg seen microscopically in skin scrapings confirms the diagnosis.

173 Lice infestation, pediculosis corporis The body louse hides and lays her eggs in the seams and crevices of clothing which must be closely examined to make the diagnosis. The patient presented with a non-specific itchy, excoriated superficial eczematous eruption on the trunk (see **44**). Since lice are rarely seen on the skin one must have a high index of suspicion for infestations and examine the clothing seams when pruritus is unexplained.

174 Pediculosis corporis, the body louse

170

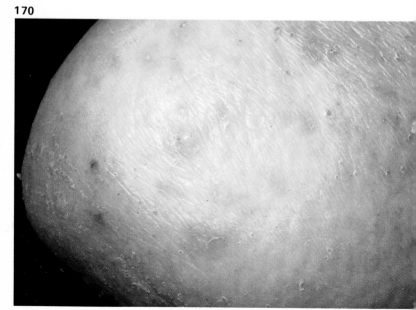

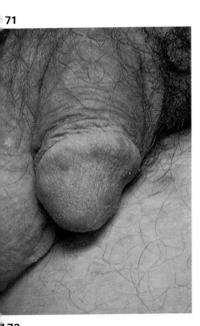

171

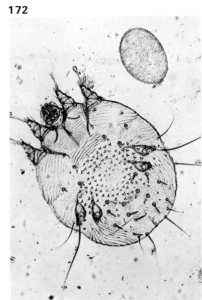

172

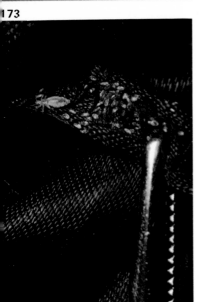

173

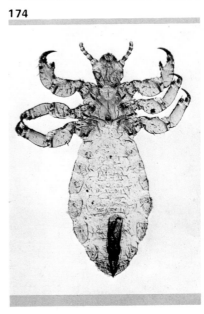

174

175 *Lice infestation, pediculosis capitis* Living lice may be hard to find but conclusive evidence of infestation is provided by 'nits', which are eggs cemented firmly to hairs. The nits give the hair a speckled appearance, particularly around the ears. The patient complained of itching on the nape and upper back. Other members of the family or cohabitants are nearly always infested and must be treated.

176 *Lice infestation, pediculosis capitis* The egg ('nit') is shown firmly cemented to the hair shaft.

177 *Pediculosis pubis, louse and nits on pubic hair* The crab-like appearance explains the popular name of the 'crab louse'. With its strong claws it grips the bases of the pubic hairs.

The patient presented with itching in the suprapubic region. These lice can be easily overlooked on casual inspection. It is necessary to examine the hair of the pubic and surrounding areas very closely with a magnifying glass if the diagnosis is not to be missed.

178 *Pediculosis pubis, the pubic louse*

175

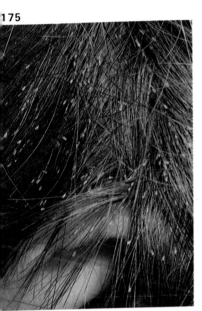

176

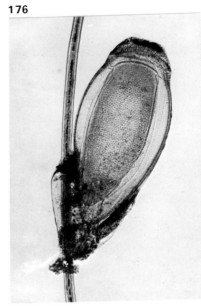

177

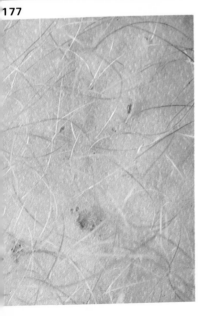

178

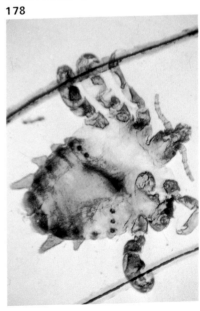

179 *Insect bites, arm* A linear or grouped distribution of bites is common. Large pruritic lesions occur only in individuals sensitized following previous bites. The presence of a central red punctum on the apex of the papule is pathognomonic for insect bites. Sometimes only one member of a family has lesions. Patients with insect bites, or the parents of affected children may be very reluctant to accept the diagnosis. The history should include enquiries into contact with animals, old furniture or strange beds. The usual agents in Britain are cat and dog fleas and bed bugs. Treatment with insecticidal cream is usually curative, but it may take several weeks before new lesions stop appearing. Sometimes lesions become granulomatous and persist for many months.

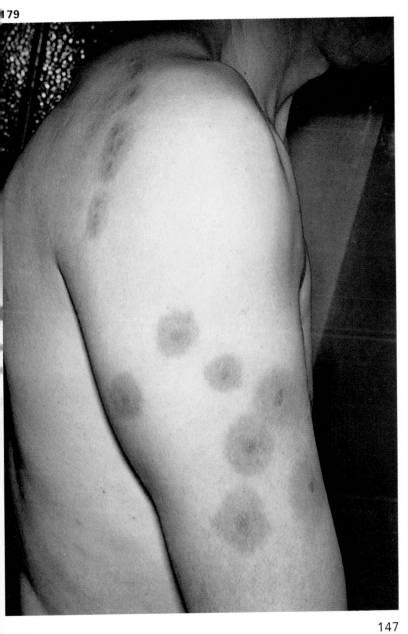

180 *Insect bites, bullous reaction* This appearance on the legs of children and young adults is commonly seen during the summer months. There is often a history of an excursion into the countryside.

181 *Creeping eruption (larva migrans), buttock* The larvae of animal parasitic worms (e.g. ankylostoma brasiliensis) are acquired by contact with beach or soil. They penetrate the skin and wander in the upper dermis producing itchy red serpentine tracks. It is a disease of inhabitants of tropical or sub-tropical climates and in those who travel there.

180

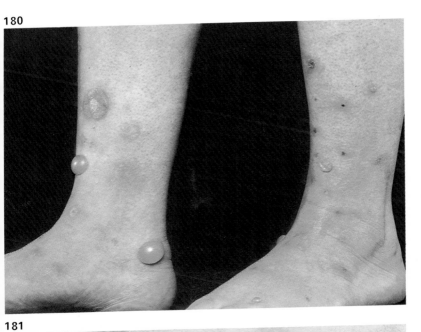

181

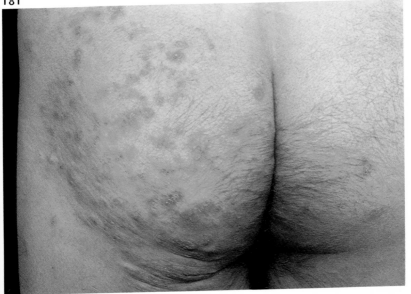

LICHEN PLANUS

This inflammatory disease of unknown cause is characterised histologically by the death of many individual epidermal cells in the germinal layer, with a heavy infiltration of lymphoid inflammatory cells in the upper dermis. The epidermis overlying the germinal layer disorder is usually thickened to produce discrete papules, but atrophy occurs in some patients. Rarely the inflammation at the dermo-epidermal junction is so intense that a subepidermal blister forms (bullous lichen planus). Hair follicles and nail matrices are sometimes destroyed by the inflammatory process.

The disease shows a very wide range of clinical appearances.

BULLOUS DISEASES

Blisters are formed when fluid collects locally in or between the layers of the skin (see page 13). Most examples seem to result from acquired inflammation (pemphigus, pemphigoid, dermatitis herpetiformis, bullous impetigo, thermal blisters), but an hereditary defect in cohesion is sometimes responsible (benign familial chronic pemphigus, epidermolysis bullosa). In pemphigus, pemphigoid and dermatitis herpetiformis are found antibodies against skin components, but their role in the pathogenesis of these diseases is not yet clear.

pemphigus **195–203**
benign familial pemphigus **204**
pemphigoid **205–208**
cicatricial pemphigoid **209–211**
dermatitis herpetiformis **212– 215**
epidermolysis bullosa **216, 217**
thermal blister **218**
herpes gestationis **219**

see also:
bullous dermatitis/eczema **29,64**
bullous impetigo contagiosa **82**
herpes simplex **152**
herpes zoster **160**
bullous fixed drug eruption **346**
porphyria **416**

182 *Lichen planus, typical chronic form, wrist flexures* Symmetrical, shiny, flat-topped, pruritic, polygonal, pinkish-mauve or violaceous papules are found on the flexor aspects of the wrists and ankles, the sacrum, shins and other areas. If the lesions are coated with a thin layer of liquid paraffin or vaseline, a net-like pattern of white streaks (Wickham's striae) may be seen ; these are pathognomonic. Healing lesions show hyperpigmentation. The buccal cavity is frequently involved.

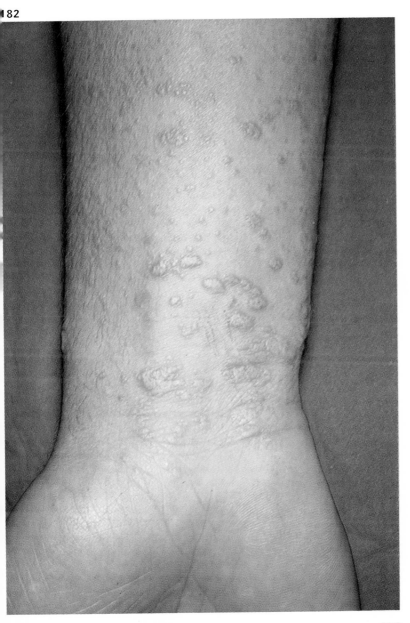

183 *Lichen planus* Extensive lesions on the lower back.

184 *Lichen planus, buccal* The insides of the cheeks show annular or reticulate white streaks. Complete examination of the mouth with torch and spatula is necessary. Sometimes white plaques or spots rather than streaks are found and rarely lesions can be ulcerated and very chronic.

185 *Lichen planus, tongue* Lesions on the tongue appear as white patches arranged longitudinally on the dorsum, as here, or in a lacy network at the margins.

186 *Lichen planus, ankle* Lesions on the lower limbs tend to be more lumpy than those on the upper limbs.

183

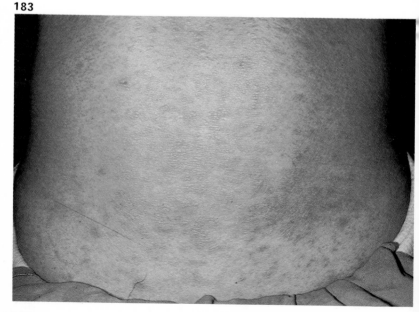

184

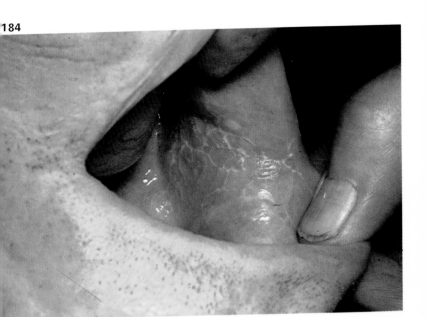

185

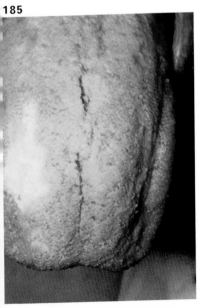

186

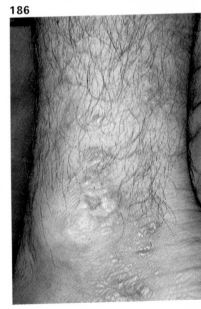

187 *Lichen planus, forearm, Negro*   In Negroes the mauvish colour cannot be seen and the lesions may look atypical. The shiny surface is still seen and hyperpigmentation is usually intense. Annular forms are common.

188 *Lichen planus, Köbner phenomenon, forearm*   Typical lesions may occur in a scratch when the disease is active.

189 *Lichen planus, glans penis*   The white lacy patterning on the corona of the glans is well shown.

190 *Lichen planus, penis*   Another pattern showing papules on the glans. Lesions also occur on the shaft of the penis and the scrotum.

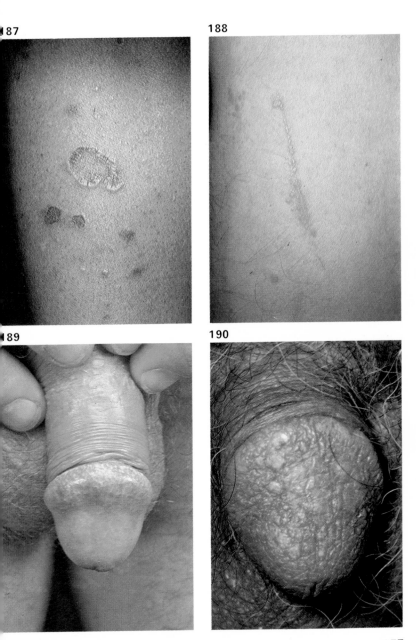

187

188

189

190

191 *Lichen planus, hypertrophic, shins* Chronic lesions on the shins are often lumpy and excoriated and the surface may have a pitted (cribriform) appearance. Hyperpigmentation assists the diagnosis.

192 *Lichen planus, nails* Irregular dystrophy of the fingernails is common when the condition has been present for a month or more. It takes the form of irregular pitting or linear streaks.

193 *Lichen planus, follicular, elbow* The inflammation can selectively involve hair follicles and destroy them.

194 *Lichen planus, follicular, scalp* Destruction of hair follicles may cause scarring alopecia.

191

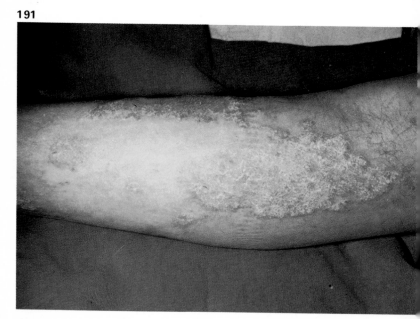

192

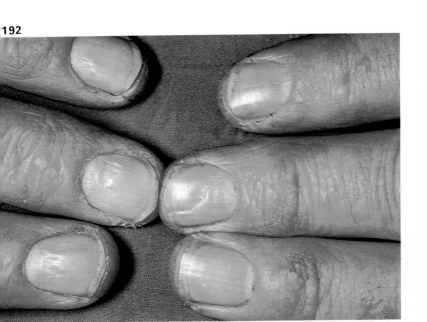

193

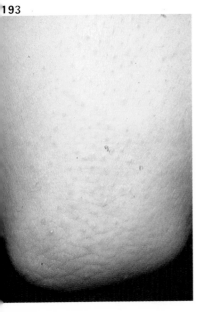

194

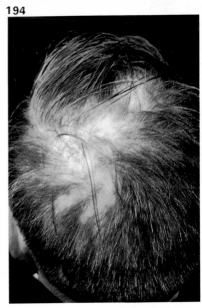

195 *Pemphigus, mouth* The mouth is involved in about 90% of cases of pemphigus and is often the first manifestation preceding skin lesions by weeks or months. Mouth lesions present as erosions or sloughs. Intact blisters are rarely seen.

196 *Pemphigus, tongue* There were irregular, very painful erosions on the tongue and floor of the mouth.

197 *Pemphigus vulgaris, back* This is usually a disease of erosions and when blisters are seen they are generally flaccid and rupture easily. Bleeding of the raw surface is common. The patient may be ill and in considerable discomfort. Skin biopsy of an early blister will show an intra-epidermal split with acantholysis. Immunofluorescent studies will demonstrate antibodies to intercellular substance in the epidermis (**203**).

195

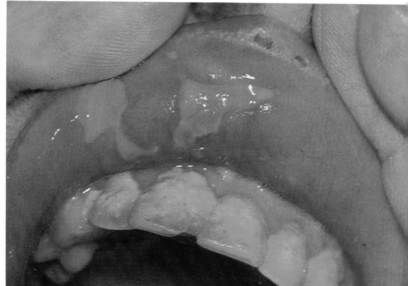

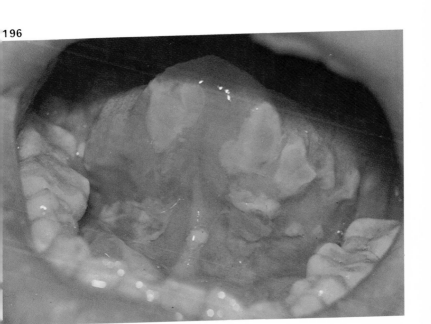

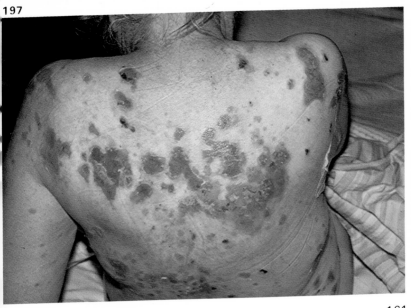

198 *Pemphigus vulgaris, trunk* A margin of ravelled epidermis around the erosions is characteristic.

199 *Pemphigus erythematosus* The first impression was that of a patchy eczema but a few small blisters were present. Skin biopsy and immunofluorescent studies are necessary to establish the diagnosis.

200 *Pemphigus, face* Lesions are eroded and crusted.

198

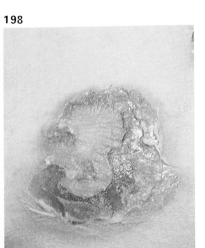

199

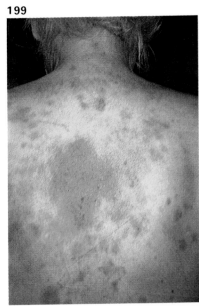

200

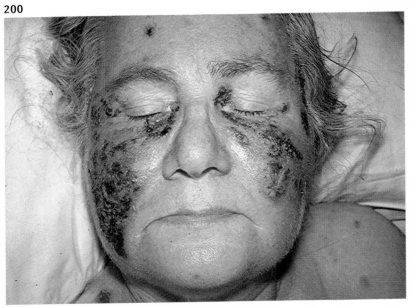

201 *Pemphigus, axilla* Lesions in flexures rapidly become macerated and infected.

202 *Pemphigus vulgaris, trunk* Small flaccid blisters are usually the first cutaneous manifestation of pemphigus but close inspection may be necessary to see them in the presence of grosser lesions. New small blisters are the best lesions to biopsy since they show the characteristic histology of an intra-epidermal blister with acantholysis.

203 *Pemphigus, indirect immunofluorescence* The patient's serum was applied to a frozen section of guinea pig lip. After washing fluorescein-labelled anti-human gamma globulin was applied. Examination by fluorescent microscopy reveals staining of the intercellular substance of the prickle-cells of the epidermis.

201

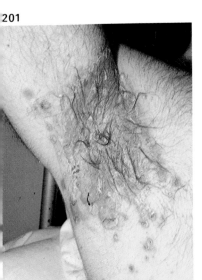

202

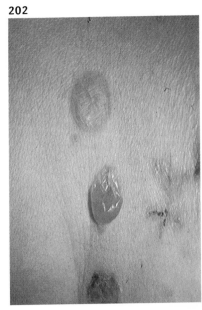

203

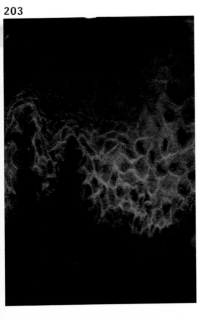

204 *Benign familial chronic pemphigus (Hailey-Hailey disease)* *submammary* This is a disease with dominant inheritance. The appearance of moist fissured erosions is typical. It usually presents as an intertrigo, especially in the groins, which is refractory to treatment. Biopsy is necessary to establish the diagnosis. Anti-epithelial antibodies are not found. Lesions do not usually appear until adult life. A family history of similar lesions is frequently obtainable.

205 *Pemphigoid, thigh* Patients are generally elderly and the disease often starts abruptly. The limbs are usually affected more than the trunk. Blisters tend to be symmetrical, large, tense and often haemorrhagic; the mouth is involved in less than 10% of cases. The patient is usually otherwise well. Skin biopsy of an early lesion will show a subepidermal blister. Immunofluorescent studies will demonstrate antibodies to the basement membrane zone of the epidermis. These antibodies are demonstrable in the lesions, in blister fluid and in serum. Lesions heal without scarring.

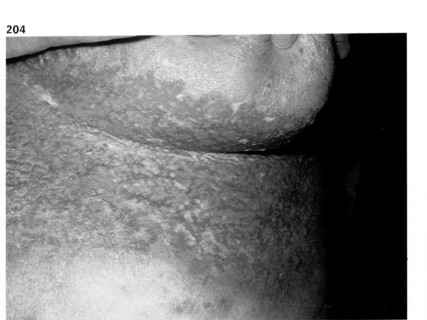

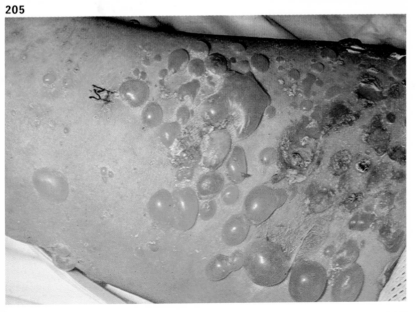

206 *Pemphigoid, forearm* Old collapsed blisters are haemorrhagic and covered with necrotic epidermis.

207 *Pemphigoid, prodromal erythema* The disease may resemble a 'toxic' erythema for weeks or months before blisters appear. A small blister is seen on the upper arm.

208 *Pemphigoid, indirect immunofluorescence* The patient's serum was incubated with a frozen section of guinea pig lip, and sites of antibody adhesion were demonstrated as in **203**. Examination in a fluorescent microscope reveals staining of the basement membrane zone at the dermo-epidermal junction.

206

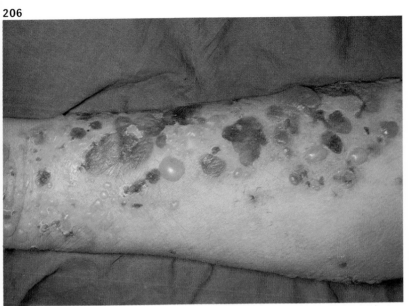

207

208

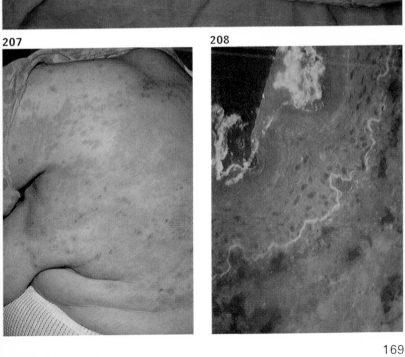

209 *Cicatricial pemphigoid (benign mucous membrane pemphigoid), intact blisters on lip* In this rare condition blisters are often recurrent at the same site and heal with scarring. Adhesions ('webs') may form in the oesophagus and give rise to dysphagia.

210 *Cicatricial pemphigoid, eye lesions* Blistering and scarring of the conjunctival sacs are serious manifestations of this disease. The patient has sore inflamed eyes; on everting the lower eyelid, adhesions between the conjunctival surfaces may be demonstrated (*synblepharons*). A single prominent adhesion is shown here.

211 *Cicatricial pemphigoid, blister, temple* Recurrent blisters in the area of the scalp may lead to scarring alopecia. Lesions around the ano-genital region are also found.

209

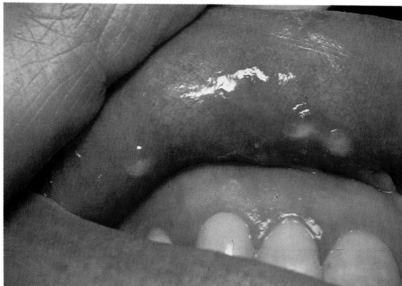

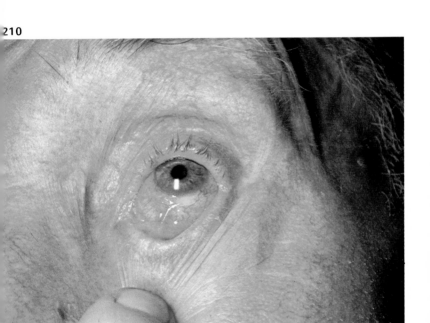

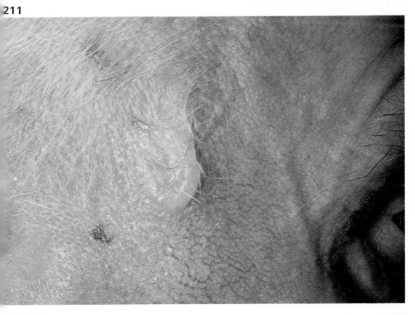

212 *Dermatitis herpetiformis, forehead* Clusters of small intensely pruritic blisters occur on the scalp, face, shoulders, lumbosacral area, the points of the elbows and the fronts of the knees. The disease may start as a 'toxic' erythema which can persist for weeks or months before blisters are seen. About two-thirds of cases have small bowel changes resembling gluten enteropathy and in these a malabsorption syndrome may be present.

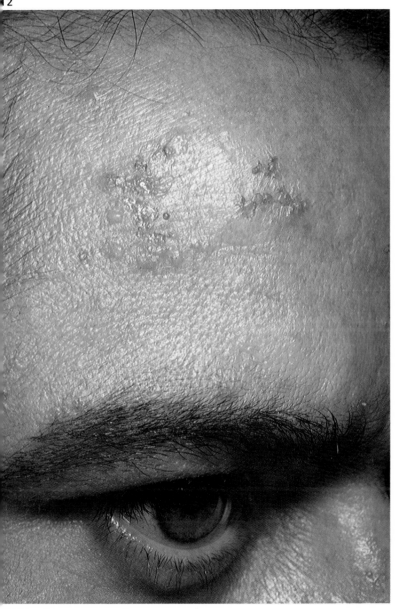

213 *Dermatitis herpetiformis, scalp and forehead* Scratching has produced small haemorrhagic crusts. Lesions may be so pruritic that the blisters are excoriated as rapidly as they are formed. This can lead to a considerable delay in making the diagnosis.

214 *Dermatitis herpetiformis, elbow* Small blisters on an erythematous background are seen.

215 *Dermatitis herpetiformis, sacral area* A common site.

213

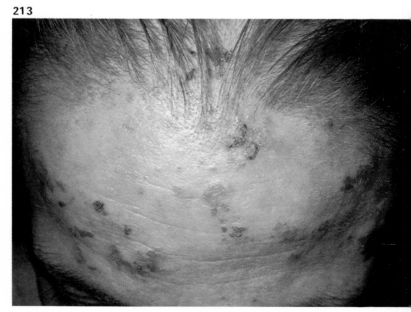

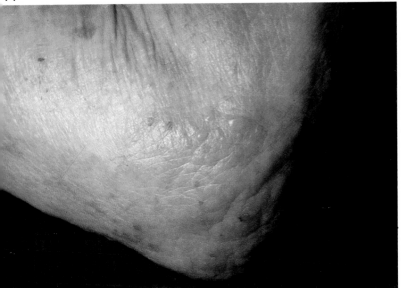

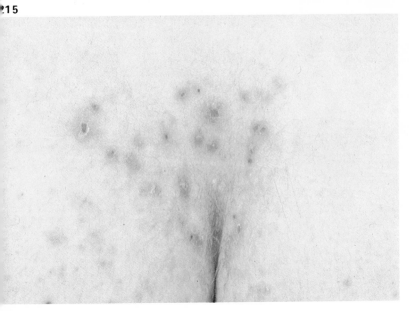

216 *Epidermolysis bullosa, plantar* In the mild form shown here blisters appear on pressure areas and at sites of trauma. Large blisters on pressure areas may be seen in patients in barbiturate coma.

217 *Epidermolysis bullosa, dystrophic, hand* Blisters form especially at sites of pressure or trauma and heal to leave scars. In this patient several fingernails have been lost.

218 *Thermal blister, shin* Caused by hot water bottle.

219 *Herpes gestationis* Best regarded as a form of pemphigoid occurring during pregnancy. Its cause is unknown. There is no evidence of viral aetiology, and it is not related to herpes simplex or herpes zoster. Onset on the lower limbs is typical. It resolves spontaneously after delivery but may recur with further pregnancies.

216

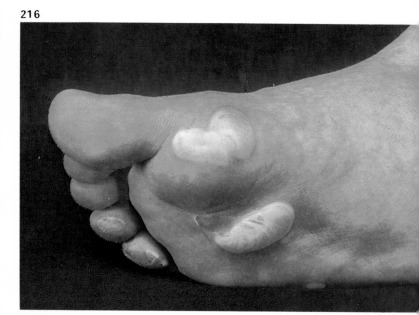

17

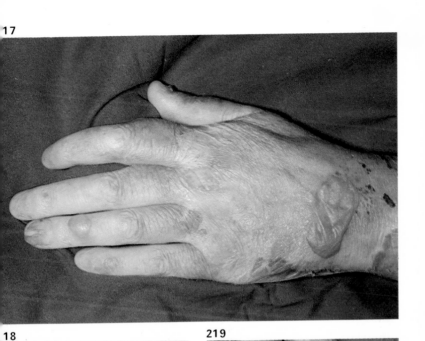

18

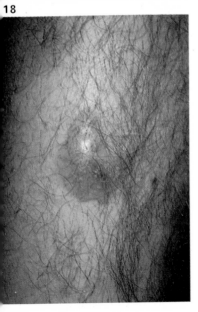

219

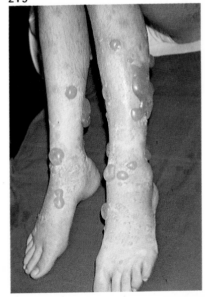

ACNE VULGARIS

A disorder in which there is hypersecretion of sebaceous glands and inflammation in hair follicles which is dependent on the presence of circulating androgenic hormones. Acne pustules contain anaerobic bacteria which are not usually regarded as pathogenic, but antibacterial agents taken systemically usually improve the disease.

ROSACEA

disorder of fair-skinned people in which there is recurrent or fixed
ythema, oedema, telangiectasia, papules and pustules affecting the
orehead, cheeks, nose and often the chin. It is a condition mostly of the
econd half of life and is associated with facial flushing. Histologically
here is oedema, vasodilatation, a predominantly lymphocytic infiltrate
nd, in advanced cases, focal granulomas with sebaceous gland hyper-
ophy. The cause is not known.

220 *Acne vulgaris, forehead* This is very common in adolescence. Features are true seborrhoea (giving skin a greasy appearance), comedones (blackheads), papules, pustules, cysts and scars.

221 *Acne vulgaris, back, close-up* Comedones block follicular orifices, a few papules and pustules are present.

222 *Acne vulgaris, cystic, face* The cysts contain pus which grows only normal skin bacteria on culture. They are often extremely tender.

223 *Acne vulgaris, scarring of back* This example is very gross, but acne is a scarring disease. Much of it is preventable with effective treatment.

220

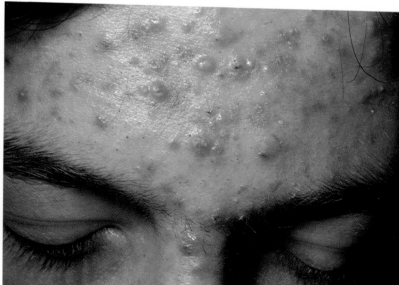

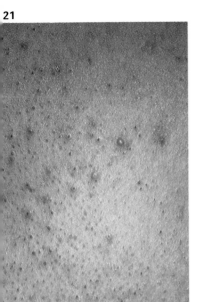

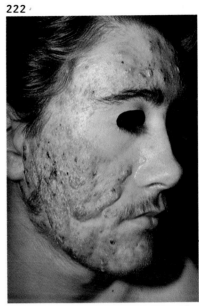

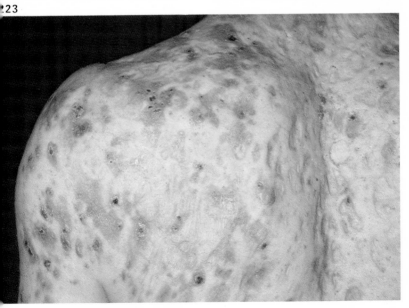

224 *Oil acne* Found on extensor surfaces of limbs in workers whose clothing becomes saturated with oil.

225 *Rosacea, face* Face shows erythema with red papules and small pustules. Blepharitis is present and some patients have sore eyes due to rosacea keratitis. Rosacea is much commoner than lupus erythematosus (see **386**, **387**) with which it is sometimes confused.

226 *Rosacea, forehead* Red papules, and pustules, are seen on a background of diffuse erythema.

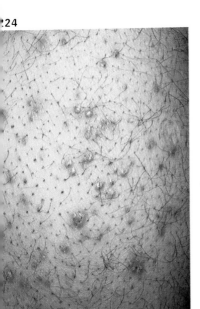

224

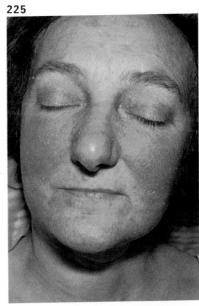

225

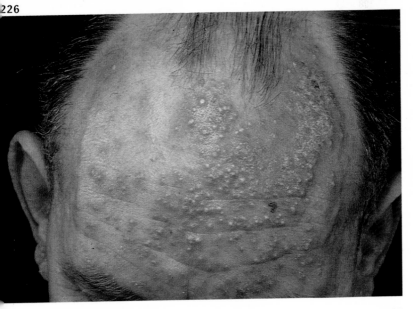

226

227 *Rhinophyma* A red swollen knobbly nose with prominent follicle mouths. A disorder of middle-aged men, it is usually associated with rosacea, and is produced by hyperplasia of sebaceous glands.

228 *Peri-oral dermatitis* A chronic red papular eruption of the lower half of the face in young women. A clear zone is seen immediately adjacent to the vermillion of the lips. It appears to be separate from eczema and rosacea and may be an effect of potent fluorinated topical steroids.

229 *Acne keloid, nape of neck* Common in Negroes. The tips of the hairs are ingrowing and keloids form. It is notoriously resistant to treatment.

227

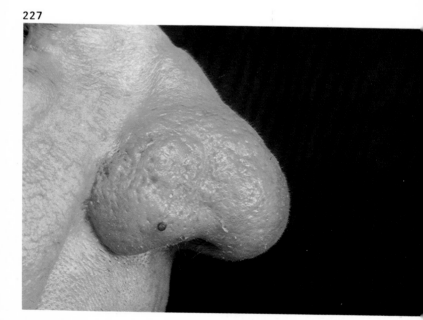

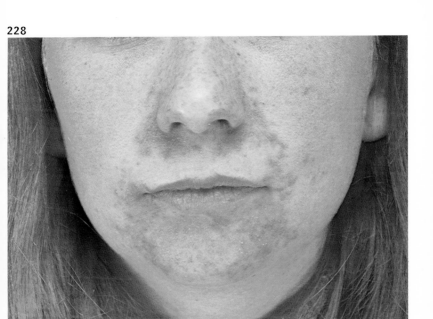

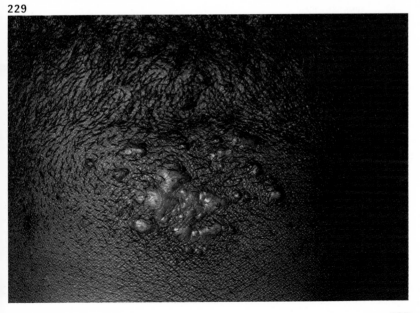

DISORDERS OF PIGMENTATION

Pigment is produced by neural crest cells (melanocytes) which normally migrate to the level of the germinal layer of the epidermis. There they manufacture melanin pigment granules which are injected into epidermal cells by means of fine dendritic processes. When melanocytes form abnormal nests in the upper dermis or at the dermo-epidermal junction the lesions are regarded as melanocytic naevi (**292–295**).

Racial pigmentation of the skin is determined by the quantity of melanin produced by melanocytes, which are present in equal numbers in all races. Perhaps the commonest form of pathological hyperpigmentation is that produced by inflammation. In the Negro skin even mild inflammation causes excessive pigment formation which may be very slow to fade.

White skin (leucoderma) occurs if melanocytes have a congenital inability to form pigment (e.g. albinism), or if they are specifically damaged by inflammation (e.g. vitiligo). Any severe inflammation may destroy pigment cells to produce a secondary leucoderma.

DISORDERS OF KERATINIZATION

In the normal skin microscopic keratin scales are being continually shed from the top of the horny layer and replaced from below. Disturbances of keratinization result from inflammation (e.g. dermatitis/eczema), friction, hereditary disorders and other unknown causes. The observable effect is the shedding of groups of dead horny cells as large scales, or the thickening of the horny layer *in situ* to produce hyperkeratosis.

230 *Mongolian spots* These non-inflammatory bluish patches are very common in Asiatics but may be seen occasionally in all nationalities. They result from aberrant melanocytes deeply situated in the dermis.

231 *Freckles (ephelides), face* These are common and not pathological. Freckles darken on exposure to sunlight. The pale skin between the freckles is very susceptible to sunburn.

232 *Freckles (ephelides), back* Profuse extra large freckles may appear in fair-skinned individuals after excessive sun exposure.

230

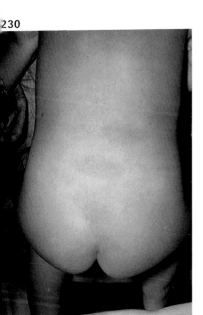

231

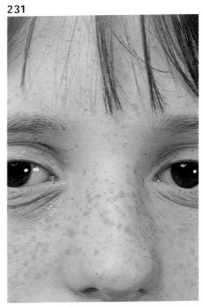

232

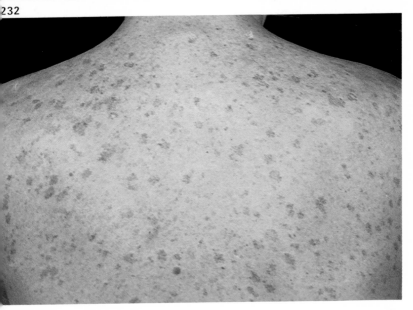

233 *Voigt's line, upper arm*   These lines, usually bilateral, are frequently found on the antero-lateral aspects of the upper arms in Negro children and young adults. They result from the developmental fusion of adjacent dermatomes with different pigmentary activity and are of no pathological significance.

234 *Pityriasis alba, face*   A common childhood disorder, of unknown cause, in which scaly hypopigmented patches are seen. They are more noticeable in dark-skinned individuals, and occur mostly on the face, but the trunk and arms may also be affected.

235 *Chloasma, face*   Patches of increased pigmentation, not always symmetrical, on the upper half of the face are very common in pregnant women. The contraceptive pill can cause a similar appearance. After delivery, or on coming off the pill, lesions fade but do not always disappear completely.

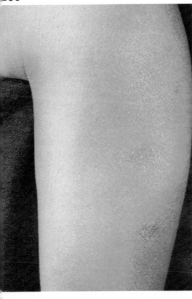

233

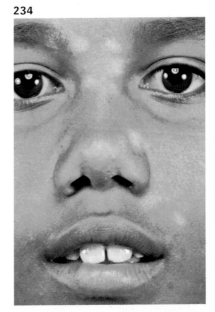

234

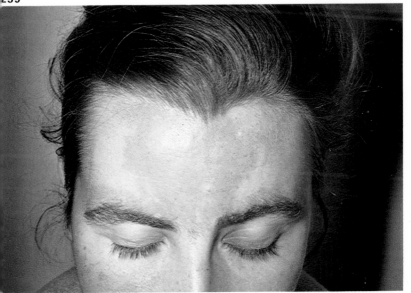

235

236 *Vitiligo* Irregular, sharply-demarcated, non-scaly, asymptomatic, symmetrical patches of complete depigmentation. Hairs in the affected area may lose their pigment. The use of Wood's light examination may show the distribution to be much more extensive than is at first obvious. Exposure to strong sunlight may be a precipitating factor. There is often a family history and it occurs more often than would be expected in association with hyperthyroidism, hypoadrenalism and Addisonian anaemia.

237 *Vitiligo* Recovery often starts by migration of viable pigment cells from hair follicles, giving rise to a stippled appearance.

236

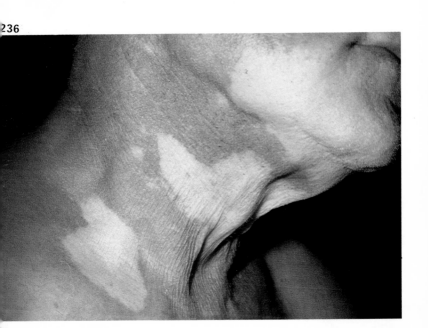

237

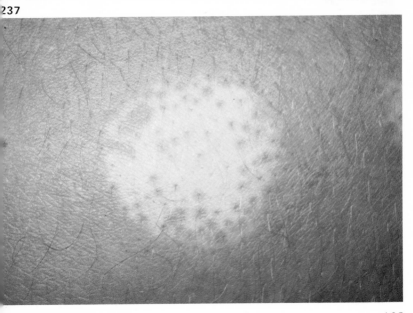

238 *Callosities, sole* Callosities are plaques of hyperkeratosis forming at sites of pressure or friction. The weight bearing areas are commonly affected, especially if there is some deformity of the foot due to bone or joint disorder. Lesions are yellowish and translucent, an appearance seen more easily if the surface is pared down with a scalpel blade. They must be distinguished from plantar viral warts (see **140, 141**).

'Corns' are nodules of hyperkeratosis, also caused by pressure or friction, which have become more deeply embedded in the skin.

239 *Soft corn, toe-web* These painful lesions are caused by pressure The hyperkeratosis is greyish-white and soft due to moisture.

240 *Tylosis, palm* There is confluent hyperkeratotic thickening of the horny layer of the palms and soles. Varieties of the condition with discrete hyperkeratosis also occur. This disorder is often familial.

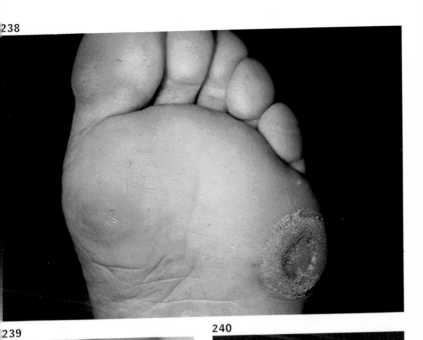

238

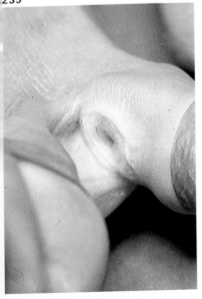

239

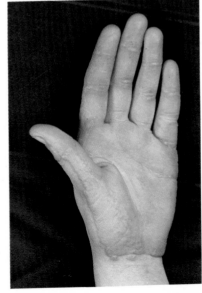

240

195

241 *Knuckle pads, hand* Thickened lesions are seen over the dorsal aspects of the finger joints. This disorder is not due to pressure or friction It is sometimes familial.

242 *Ichthyosis vulgaris, trunk* A familial disorder of dominant inheritance. The skin is very dry and scaly. Typical features are the brownish patterning of hyperkeratosis, and the dry scaly nipples. The flexures tend to be spared.

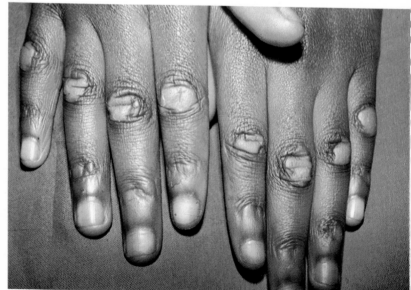

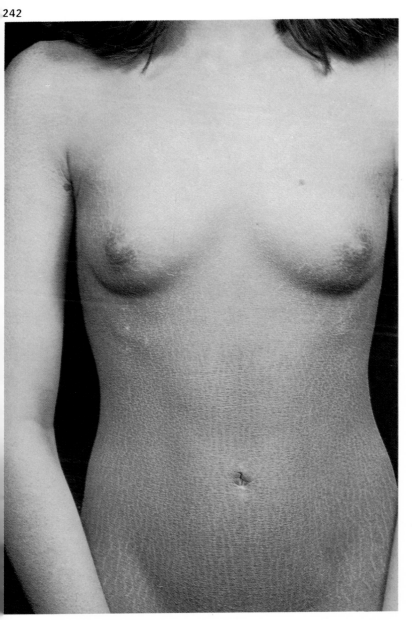

243 *Darier's disease, chest* A dominant familial disorder. Profuse symmetrical small warty brown or brownish-red papules are seen on the neck and upper trunk. There can be exacerbations and remissions for no obvious reason.

244 *Darier's disease, pitting of palps of fingers* This is a useful confirmatory sign of Darier's disease. There are numerous tiny pits in the palp skin, interrupting the normal ridge pattern of finger prints.

245 *Darier's disease, fingernails* V-shaped nicks in the free edges of the nails are seen.

243

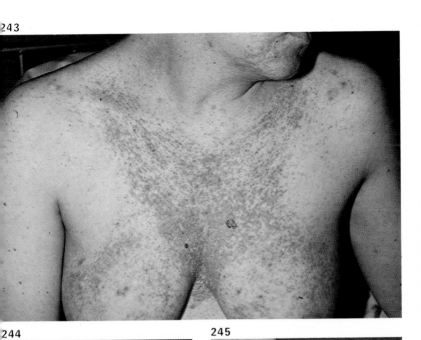

244

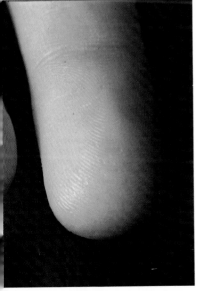

245

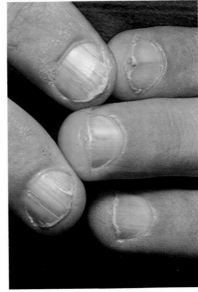

246 *Pityriasis rubra pilaris, abdomen* A rare condition characterised by red scaly plaques and follicular papules. It is sometimes very extensive and can be a cause of erythroderma. It may look very like
psoriasis but can usually be distinguished from it by the characteristic
follicular lesions, the appearance of the palms and soles, and small
islands of normal skin in otherwise homogeneous plaques.

247 *Pityriasis rubra pilaris, palms* There is orange-coloured diffuse
hyperkeratosis ; scaling is confined to the palmar flexures. The soles are
often similarly affected and the keratin may be very thick.

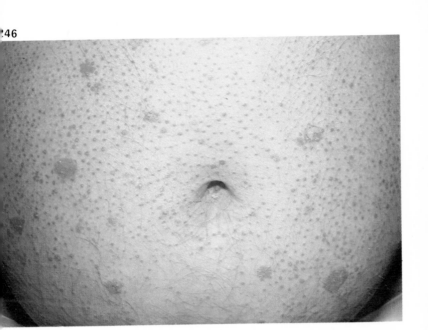

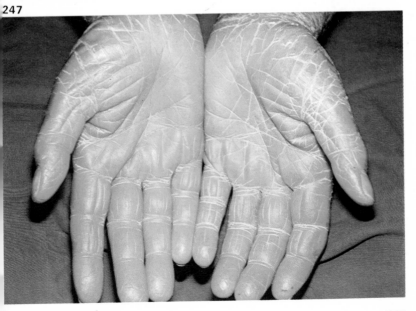

248 *Pityriasis capitis ('dandruff')* Fine greasy scales are seen. The whole surface of the scalp is affected and there is usually no erythema, thus distinguishing it from psoriasis.

Pityriasis capitis may be associated with acne vulgaris (**216**), seborrhoeic dermatitis (**51**) and seborrhoeide (**56**).

249 *Keratosis pilaris* This is a very common disorder. The characteristic site is the posterior aspect of the upper arm. The hair follicles are plugged with keratin and there is often, as here, an associated punctate erythema.

250 *Keratosis pilaris, close-up*

248

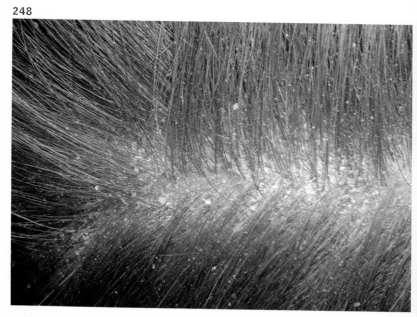

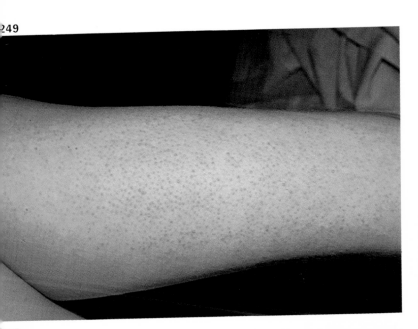

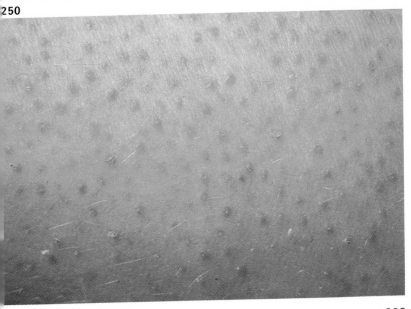

HAIR DISORDERS

NAIL DISORDERS

251 *Ingrowing hairs* Common in Negroes in the beard area. The shaved hairs curl back into the skin and small inflammatory papules arise. Sometimes there is also keloid formation.

252 *Alopecia areata* This is common in childhood and in young adults, but occurs at all ages. One or more round or oval smooth bald patches appear. Redness, swelling, broken hairs and scaling, features of scalp ringworm, are absent. Although most commonly seen on the scalp, the beard and other areas may be affected.

253 *Alopecia areata, adult* Two adjacent patches are seen.

251

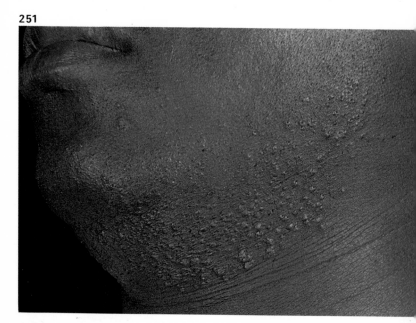

52

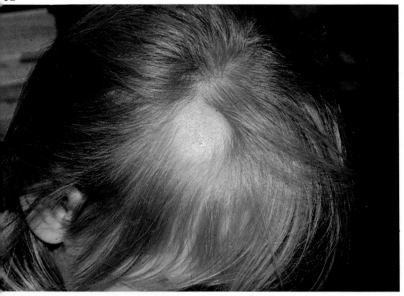

53

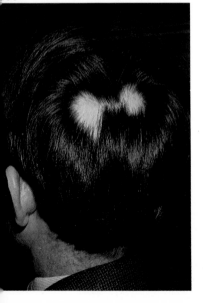

207

254 *Alopecia areata, 'exclamation mark' hairs* At the margins of active lesions are found short hairs which are of normal width at the tip and narrow at the base. They are pathognomonic. In some patients diffuse coarse pitting of the fingernails is found.

255 *Alopecia areata* White regrowth is common. It may darken later.

256 *Alopecia totalis* This is the end result of very severe alopecia areata. If all body hair is lost it is termed alopecia universalis. This patient also has a prominent 'naevus flammeus' of the nape, a commonly found type of capillary haemangioma (**377**) ; the association with alopecia is fortuitous.

257 *Alopecia areata, beard* Bald patches in the beard area and in other normally hairy areas on the body may be observed.

254

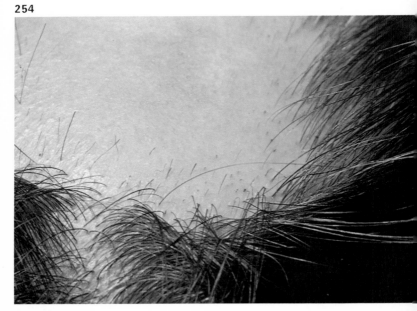

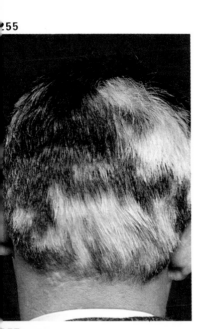

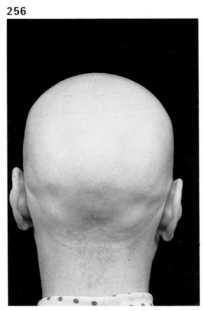

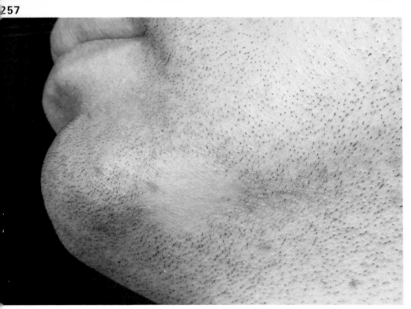

258 *Alopecia due to hair pulling (trichotillomania)* A hair pulling neurosis. The hair is short in affected areas of the scalp but all the follicles are filled and no scalp disease is seen. Adults usually admit to hair pulling. It is also seen in children, but their parents may be loath to accept that it is self-inflicted.

259 *Alopecia, diffuse, due to cytotoxic therapy* Diffuse alopecia is common during cytotoxic therapy. Other chemicals which may produce a similar picture are heparinoid and coumarin anticoagulants, antithyroid drugs, thallium salts and hypervitaminosis A.

Endocrine disturbances can also produce diffuse alopecia, e.g. normal pregnancy, hypothyroidism, hyperthyroidism, hypoparathyroidism, hypopituitary states and poorly controlled diabetes mellitus. Patchy hair loss may be found in secondary syphilis.

260 *Alopecia, scarring (cicatricial)* Intense dermal inflammation can destroy hair follicles and give rise to scarring. Possible causes are lupus erythematosus, lichen planus, scleroderma and severe fungal and bacterial infections. Biopsy of the edge of an active area is indicated. If no cause is found the term 'pseudopelade' is often used.

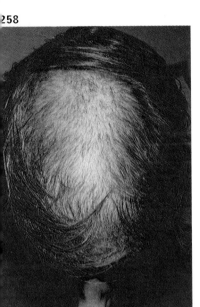

258

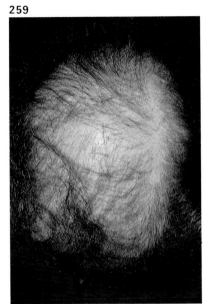

259

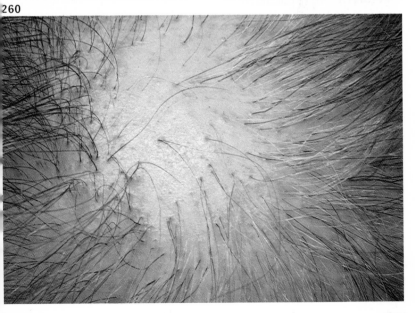

260

261 *Follicular mucinosis* Raised red plaques with loss of hair. There is inflammation round the hair follicles with degeneration of their epithelium, which accumulate mucin within them. It may be associated with a cutaneous reticulosis. The face, scalp, neck and shoulders are the most common sites.

262 *Alopecia, traction* Repeated traction (e.g. by curlers or hot combs) can result in temporary or permanent loss of hair.

261

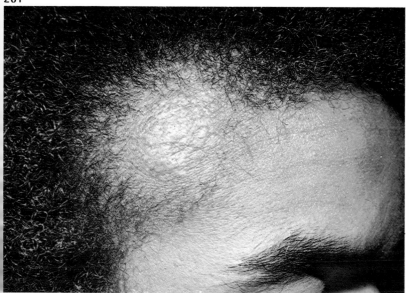

262

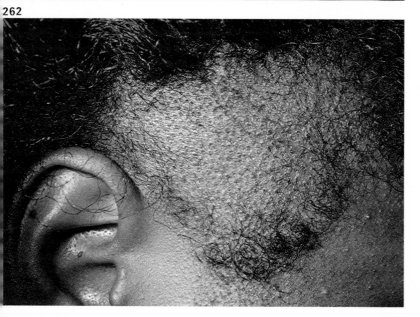

263 *Dermatitis/eczema, nail dystrophy* Any form of eczema of the dorsal fingers extending to the nail fold can produce nail dystrophy.

264 *Nail dystrophy, traumatic* An injury to the nail fold can cause permanent subsequent nail dystrophy.

265 *Nail dystrophy, traumatic* Habitual 'picking' of the nail fold causes an irregular dystrophy which is reversible when the habit ceases.

263

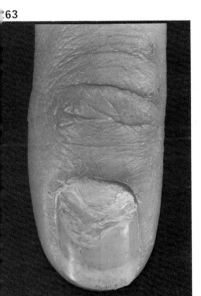

264

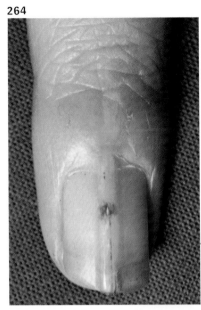

265

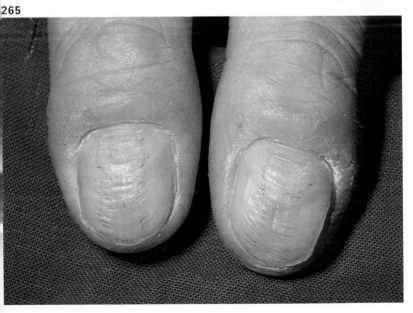

215

266 *Striate leuconychia* Transverse white lines, due to manicuring, appeared in this case. They can also arise for no obvious reason.

267 *Beau's lines, fingernails* There are transverse depressions affecting all the nails symmetrically. They occur as a result of temporary disturbance of nail growth during an acute debilitating illness (e.g. coronary thrombosis, pneumonia and acute infectious fevers). The depressions move distally as normal nail growth is resumed. Normal fingernails grow at the rate of 0·5 to 1·2 mm per week and one can conclude by inspection that this patient had an acute illness two to three months previously.

268 *Ingrowing toenail* The lateral nail fold is penetrated by the edge of the curved nail plate to produce pain, sepsis and, after a time, granulations. Tight shoes are the most common predisposing cause.

266

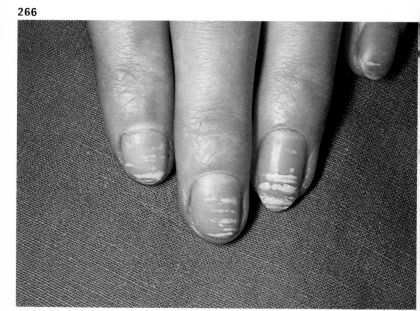

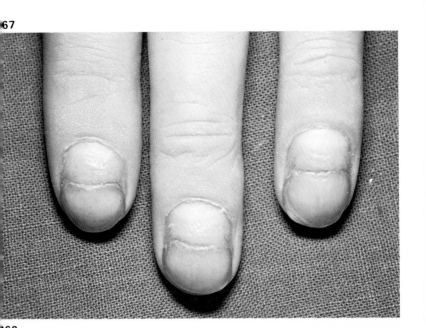

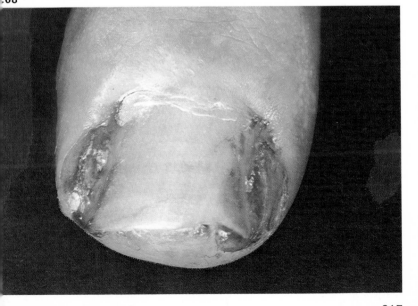

269 *Median nail dystrophy* A characteristic 'fir-tree' appearance, often bilateral. Of unknown cause it may resolve and recur for no apparent reason.

270 *Nails, splinter haemorrhage* Small haemorrhages at the free margin of the nail are common in individuals doing heavy manual work. More proximal lesions may indicate septicaemia.

271 *Yellow nail syndrome* Slowly growing thickened yellow nails excessively curved both longitudinally and laterally are associated with peripheral lymphoedema. Bronchiectasis, pleural effusion and lymphoedema elsewhere may be present. It often starts in middle age. The underlying disorder is a lymphatic vessel abnormality, often hypoplasia.

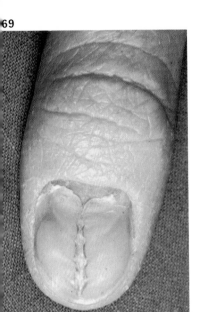

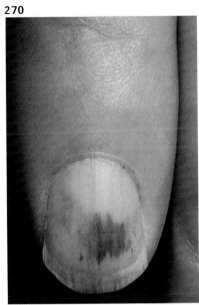

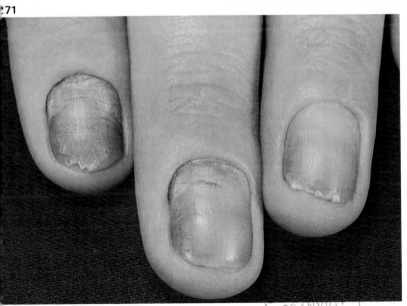

TONGUE AND MOUTH DISORDERS

272 *Tongue, furred* Furring may occur in oral or upper respiratory infections and in fevers. Heavy smoking is also a factor. It is due to hypertrophy of the filiform papillae or impairment of normal desquamation.

273 *Black tongue* A black 'hairy' tongue can be produced after antibiotic ingestion or for no known reason. It is often chronic.

274 *Median rhomboid glossitis* Lesions may be smooth or thickened. It occurs in adults and is not pre-cancerous.

275 *Geographical tongue* A benign inflammatory disorder of unknown cause. The pattern can change rapidly.

272

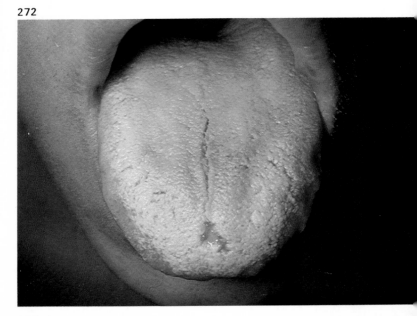

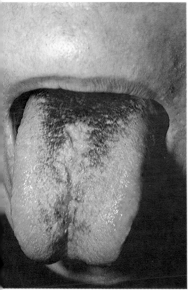

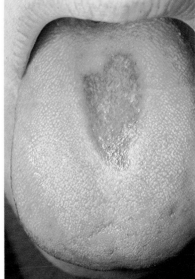

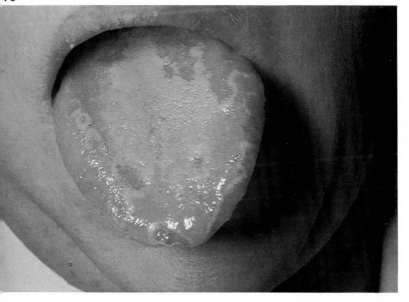

276 *Smooth tongue* The smooth red glossy appearance is due to loss of papillae. It is sore. Possible causes are anaemias (iron deficiency or megaloblastic), vitamin deficiencies, malabsorption syndromes and antibiotic ingestion.

277 *Aphthous ulcers, tongue* Painful ulcers arise on the tongue or anterior buccal mucosa. They can be recurrent even in otherwise healthy individuals.

278 *Vincent's stomatitis* There is a characteristic 'foetor oris' which can give the diagnosis before inspection. Superficial red erosions around the teeth are seen. The infection may complicate other buccal diseases such as pemphigus vulgaris. Smears from lesions show *Borrelia vincenti* (Vincent's spirochaete) and *Bacillus fusiformis*.

276

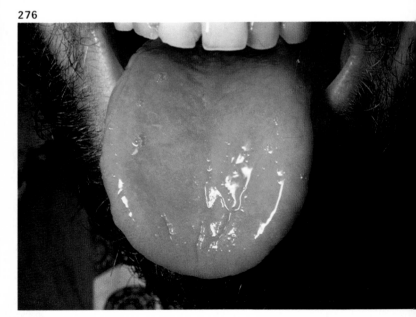

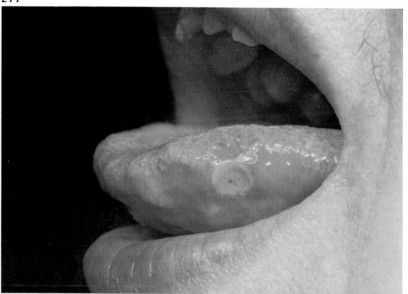

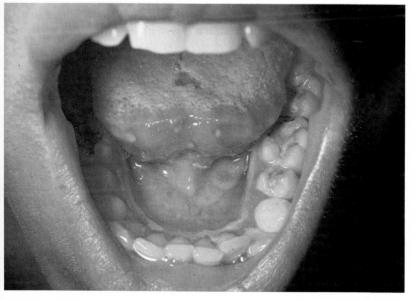

TUMOURS

Benign

Pre-malignant

Malignant

279 *Skin tags, neck* These are small raised soft smooth papillomas covered with normal or slightly hyperpigmented skin. Common in middle-aged women, especially on the sides of the neck and axillae.

280 *Keloid, upper arm* Overgrowth of connective tissue in a scar is particularly common in Africans. The tendency is enhanced if foreign matter is introduced. A keloid vaccination scar is shown. It persists, in contrast to a hypertrophic scar.

281 *Keloid, ear lobe* This is a complication of ear piercing, particularly if followed by bacterial infection.

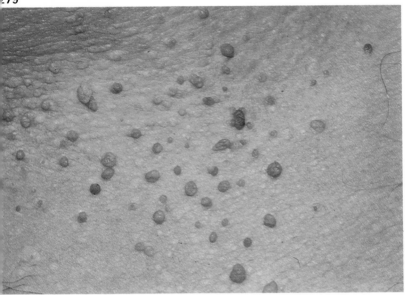

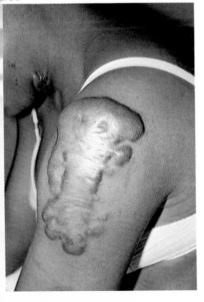

282 *Sebaceous cyst (tricholemmal cyst), scalp* One or more are common in the scalp of adults. They are firm when small but large lesions tend to be soft or even fluctuant. They contain keratin and its breakdown products. They may become infected and suppurate.

283 *Sebaceous cysts (epidermoid cysts), scrotum* It is possible to excise these lesions, but new ones continue to appear.

284 *Histiocytoma (dermatofibroma), shin* A hard dome-shaped nodule with a smooth or slightly scaly surface forms. Often a narrow rim of hyperpigmentation is present around the nodule. Multiple lesions on the legs and thighs are common in middle age.

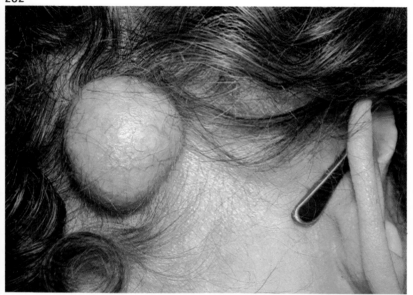

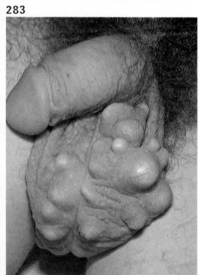

284

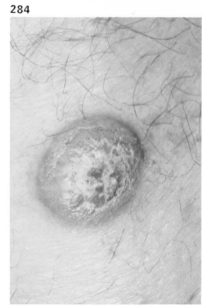

285 *Milia, cheek* These small hard white papules are dense keratin cysts in the upper dermis. They occur spontaneously, especially on the cheeks, and at the sites of healed blisters.

286 *Dermatosis papulosa nigra, cheek* These small black soft warty growths resemble seborrhoeic warts, and are commonly seen on the face in Negroes.

287 *Warty epidermal naevus, back of neck* These lesions are either congenital or appear in the first decade of life. Long linear lesions can occur on the limbs (naevus unius lateralis). Excision is the best treatment.

288 *'Seborrhoeic' wart* Soft greasy warty lesions, often pigmented and hyperkeratotic. Found on the trunk and elsewhere in people of middle age and above. May be single or very numerous. One of the commonest benign skin tumours in the elderly.

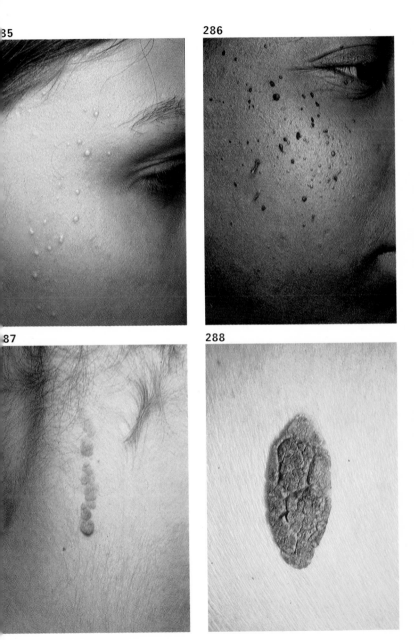

289 *'Seborrhoeic' wart, temple* The temple is a common site for large lesions. They do not become malignant and are easily treated by curettage and electrocautery.

290 *'Seborrhoeic' warts, abdomen* Numerous lesions were seen on the trunk of a very old lady.

291 *Sebaceous naevus (naevus sebaceus of Jadassohn), scalp* A circumscribed plaque of densely packed yellowish papules. They are either present at birth or develop during childhood. They become thicker with age. Excision is the treatment of choice.

289

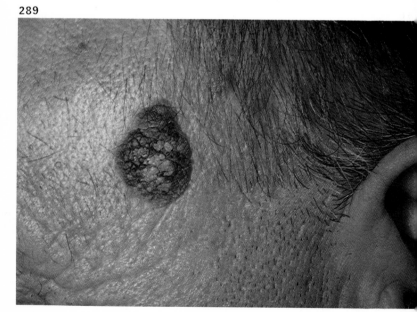

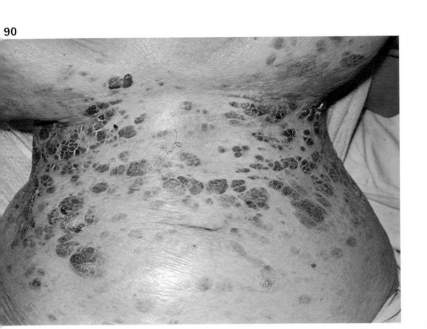

90

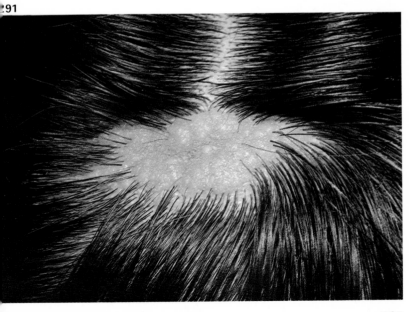

291

292, 293 & 294 *Melanocytic naevus ('mole')* These lesions are macules or soft to firm nodules which may vary in pigmentation from pale skin colour to deepest black. They become noticeable around puberty and tend to grow very slowly during adult life. They occur particularly on the face and trunk and are so common that practically every individual has several of them. In these and in other pigmented lesions rapid increase in size, spreading pigmentation, bleeding or ulceration may indicate change to malignant melanoma and urgent complete surgical excision with immediate histological examination is indicated.

292

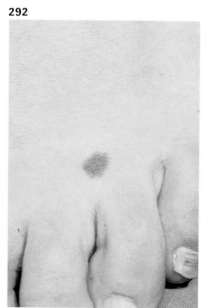

293

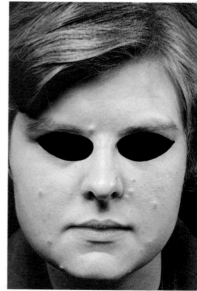

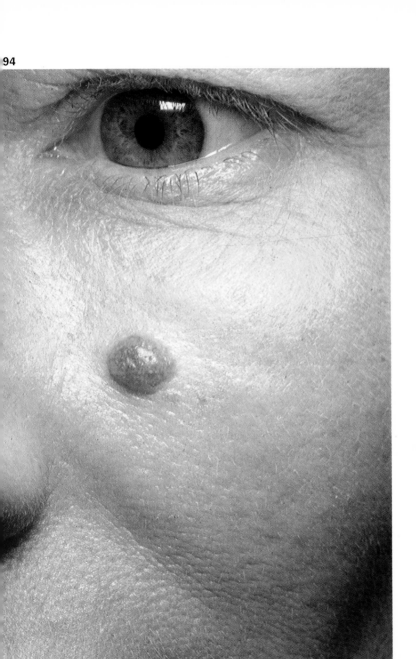

295 *Melanocytic naevus, trunk*

296 *Halo naevus, trunk (Sutton's naevus; leucoderma acquisitum centrifugum)* Occurs mostly on the trunk in children and young adults. The central nodule is usually a benign pigmented melanocytic naevus.

297 *Juvenile melanoma, cheek* A reddish or brownish smooth or rough nodule found most commonly on the face or legs of children. It is clinically benign but histologically it may closely resemble a malignant melanoma.

298 *Blue naevus, scalp margin* The deep blue colour is due to the optical effect of collections of pigment cells deep in the dermis. It persists unchanged. Malignant transformation is very rare.

295

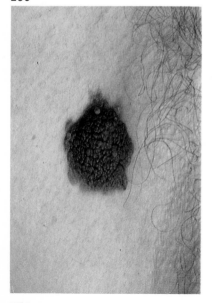

296

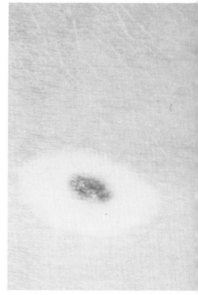

97

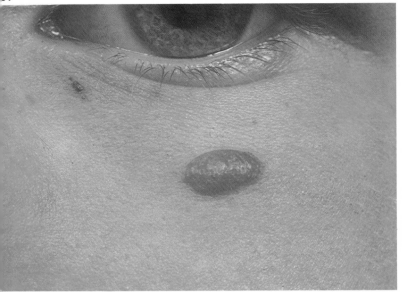

98

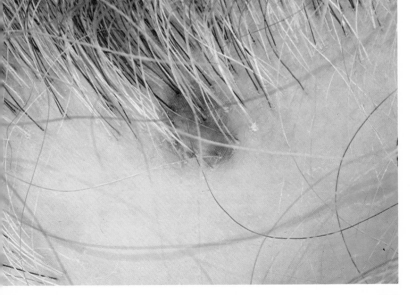

299 & 300 *Pyogenic granuloma (granuloma telangiectaticum)*
A rapidly developing benign proliferation of granulation tissue sometimes at the site of minor trauma. It is red and friable and bleeds easily.
The base is often pedunculated and surrounded by a collar of thickened
epithelium. In the palmar lesion the keratin collar has been lifted and
reflected over the granuloma to make it visible.

301 *Pigmented hairy epidermal naevus (Becker's naevus)*
Usually starting at puberty, it appears in the shoulder or chest region and
remains static during adult life. Hairs may be coarser than normal in the
lesion. It occurs mostly in men.

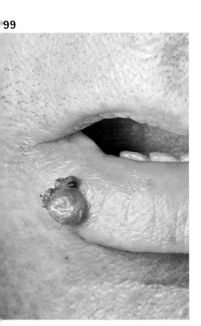

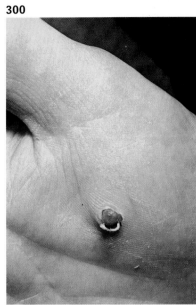

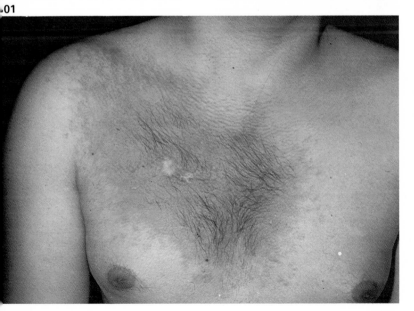

302 *Hairy pigmented naevus, sacrum* This lesion is present at birth and grows with the child. There may be underlying vertebral column abnormality (spina bifida).

303 *Adenoma sebaceum, face* These hamartomas of connective tissue are a cutaneous marker of tuberous sclerosis (epiloia). One should ask about a personal or family history of epileptic fits. Periungual fibromas and rough 'shagreen patches' in the lumbar area may also be present

304 *Periungual fibromas* These lesions, which may affect fingers or toes, are closely associated with adenoma sebaceum in epiloia (tuberous sclerosis). Isolated lesions, as here, are also seen.

302

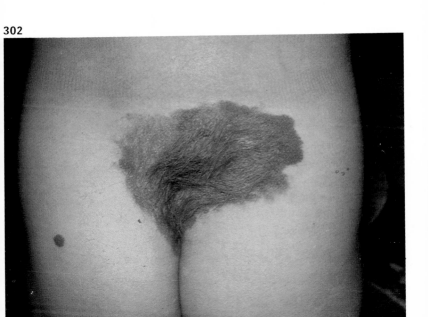

303

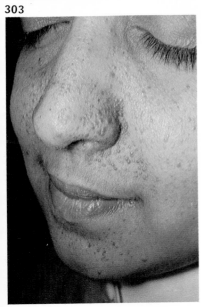

304

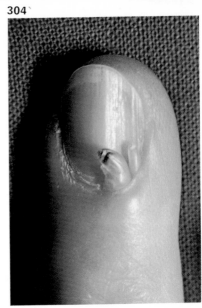

305 *Neurofibromatosis (Von Recklinghausen's disease),*
axilla Numerous symmetrical, soft, often pigmented tumours associated
with 'café-au-lait' macules. Freckling of axilla is characteristic.

306 *Neurofibroma, chin* Solitary neurofibromas usually occur on the
face. They are very soft tumours.

307 *Urticaria pigmentosa (mastocytosis), child* Brownish
macules which urticate on friction, due to accumulations of mast cells
in the upper dermis. Bone lesions may occur. The childhood form usually
resolves spontaneously after several years.

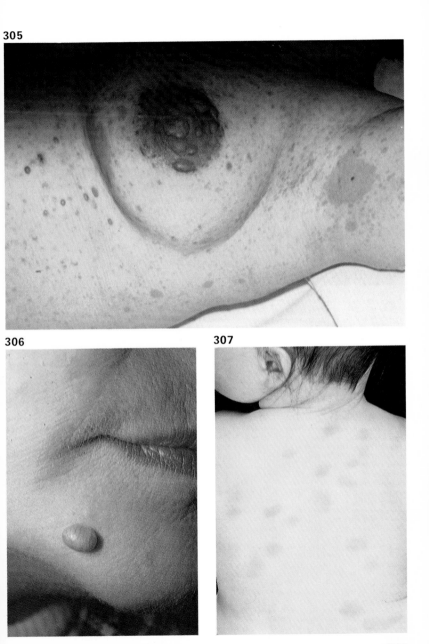

305

306

307

245

308 *Urticaria pigmentosa, thigh, adult*   The brownish macules have been rubbed to produce reddish urticating papules. Significant bone and visceral lesions may occur in adults.

309 *Keratoacanthoma (molluscum sebaceum), neck*   A rapidly growing globular tumour found mostly in light-exposed areas in middle-aged individuals. It starts as a papule and attains its maximum size in four to eight weeks. Its symmetrical shape and crateriform plug of keratin distinguishes it, in most cases, from a squamous carcinoma which it may resemble both clinically and histologically.

310 *Keratoacanthoma, cheek*   A later lesion than in **309**. If un-treated, the keratin plug is extruded and the lesion involutes to leave a ragged depressed scar. Treatment by excision or by curettage and cautery usually gives a better cosmetic result than that obtained by allowing it to resolve spontaneously.

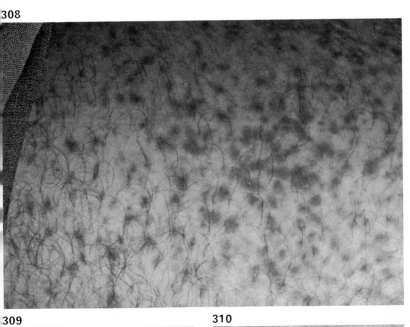

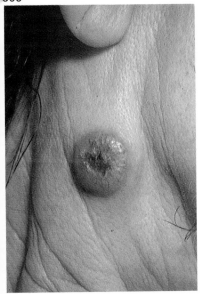

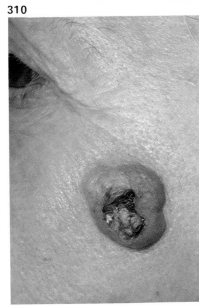

311 *Bowen's disease, shin* A dull red sharply marginated patch with irregular keratin crusting. If the crust is removed a moist granulating oozing surface is seen. The lesion is premalignant and can be regarded as a squamous *carcinoma-in-situ*. It is associated with internal carcinoma in a proportion of cases and there may be a history of previous inorganic arsenic ingestion.

312 *Solar keratosis, cheek and nose* Small irregular warty plaques with tough adherent scales. Hard accretions of keratin forming a 'cutaneous horn' may be seen as in the lesion on the cheek ; some turn into squamous carcinoma. Patients are fair-skinned and usually have had excessive exposure to sunlight, the lesions appearing in light-exposed areas. Solar keratoses are particularly common in Australia, South Africa and the southern United States.

311

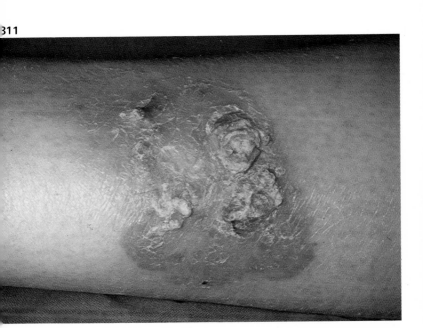

312

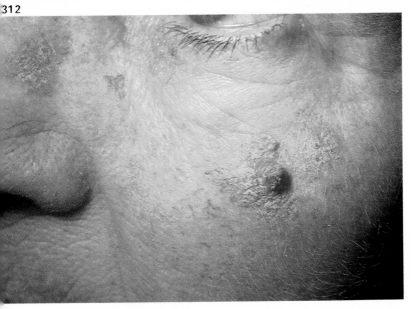

313 *Arsenical keratoses, fingers* Multiple corn-like lesions on the palms and fingers occur in patients with a past history of ingestion of inorganic arsenic, often decades before.

314 *Lentigo of Hutchinson (melanotic freckle, melanosis circumscripta preblastomatosa)* The cheek of elderly people is the most common site. It is solitary, flat and dark, and grows by very slow extension. It may be regarded as a *melanoma-in-situ.* Some lesions develop a malignant melanoma, which has a better prognosis than is usual with this tumour.

315 *Leukoplakia, lip* Lesions are soft, thickened and white, often with a mosaic-patterned surface. The lower lip, oral mucosa and vulva are the usual sites. Transformation into squamous carcinoma is not uncommon.

313

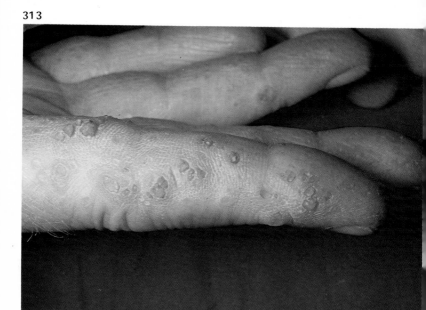

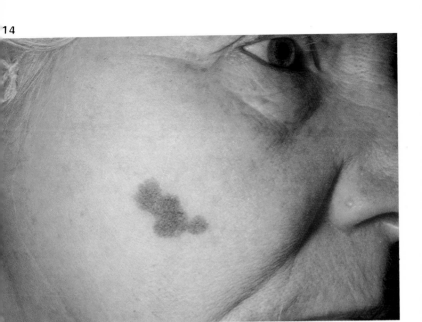

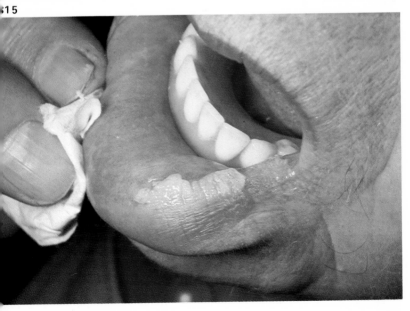

316 *Malignant melanoma, chest* An ulcerated black nodule with surrounding irregular spreading pigmentation. This is surgical emergency. Lesions may arise in a pre-existing pigmented melanocytic naevus, in a patch of melanosis or without a preceding lesion.

317 *Malignant melanoma, toe-web* An ulcerated sloughing pigmented plaque of recent onset.

318 *Malignant melanoma, cheek* A non-ulcerated nodule showing only slight pigmentation.

319 *Malignant melanoma, amelanotic, thumb* Friable granulations are seen. If pigment is present the term 'melanotic whitlow' is often used.

316

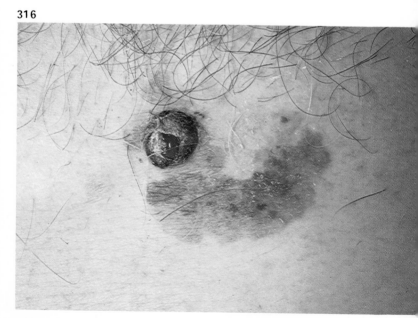

17

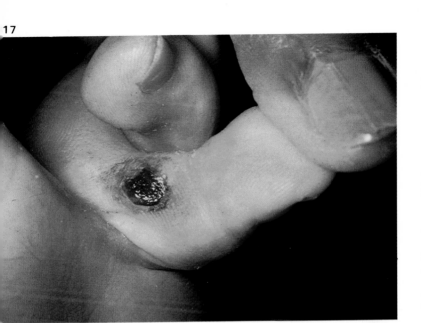

18

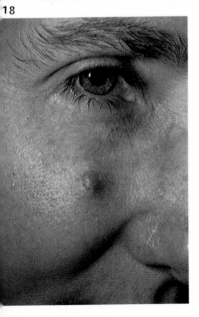

319

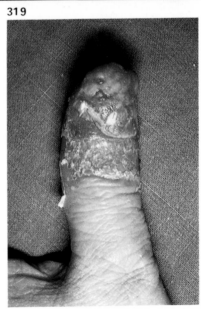

253

320 *Basal cell carcinoma, ulcerated* One or more clustered pearly nodules with associated telangiectasia and early ulceration ('rodent ulcer'). The majority are found on the forehead or face and are associated with previous prolonged light exposure.

321 *Basal cell carcinoma, early lesion, lower eyelid* A single hard translucent nodule with telangiectases on the surface.

322 *Basal cell carcinoma, pigmented, forehead* Minor degrees of pigmentation are not uncommon. A heavily pigmented lesion may be difficult to distinguish from a malignant melanoma.

323 *Basal cell carcinoma, advanced* Neglected lesions can be very destructive.

320

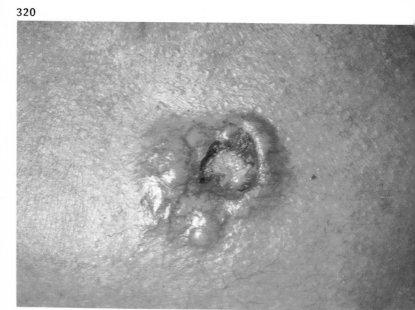

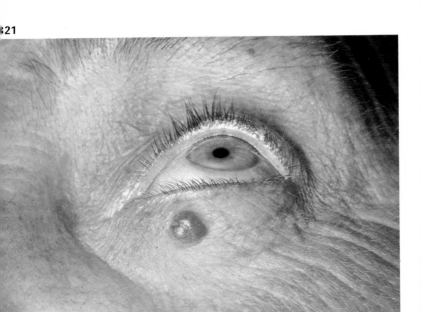

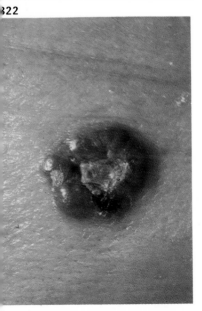

323

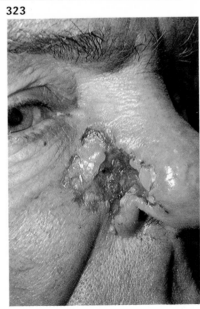

324 *Basal cell carcinoma, superficial, back* Multiple flat lesions may be associated with past ingestion of inorganic arsenic. The translucent nodular raised edge indicated the diagnosis.

325 *Squamous cell carcinoma, lower lip* An ulcerated lesion with hard raised edges. The lower lip is a common site, associated with previous excessive light exposure and cigarette or pipe smoking.

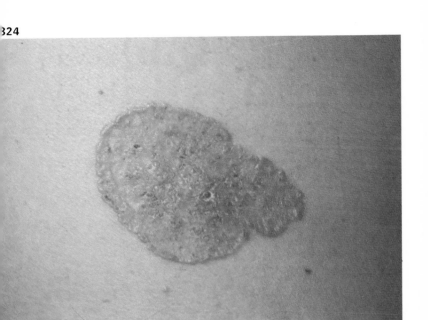

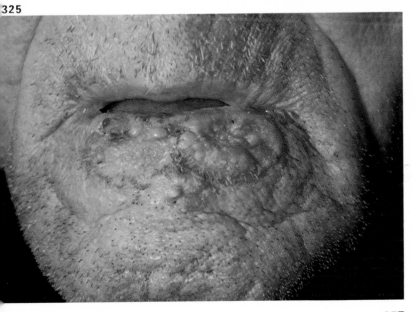

326 *Squamous carcinoma, forehead* Solar keratoses are present. The squamous tumour grew very rapidly.

327 *Squamous carcinoma, root of ear* The lesion arose in an old scar of lupus erythematosus. Similar lesions may arise in scars due to lupus vulgaris or x-rays.

328 *Mycosis fungoides, buttocks* Lesions appear as one or more well-circumscribed, usually pruritic, dark red or brownish scaly plaques. They grow slowly over a period of years and new ones appear. Histology shows a heavy dermal inflammatory infiltrate with large malignant ('mycosis') cells invading the epidermis.

326

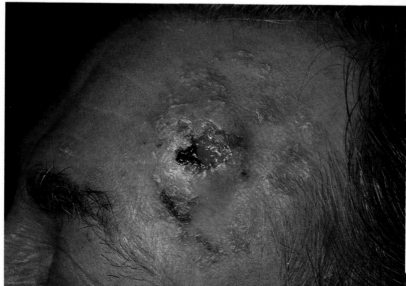

327

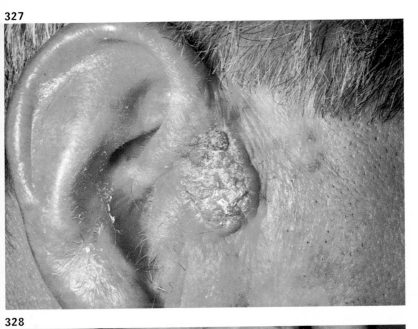

328

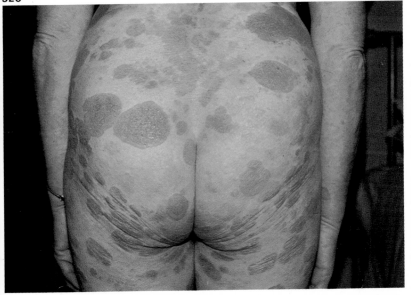

329 *Mycosis fungoides, thigh* Sometimes lesions are diffuse with atrophy, reticulate pigmentation and telangiectasia ('poikiloderma').

330 *Mycosis fungoides, chest* In the late stage, which may be decades after the onset, ulcerating tumorous nodules appear in the plaques.

331 *Paget's disease of the nipple* A red scaly lesion with a sharply marginated, slowly advancing edge. It is always associated with an intraduct mammary carcinoma and, histologically, malignant cells can be seen invading the epidermis.

329

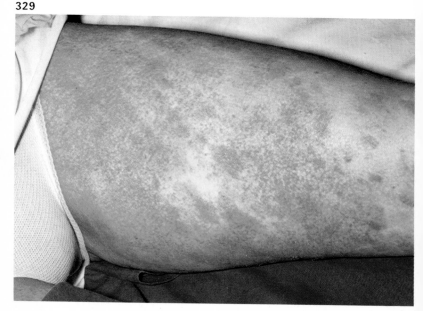

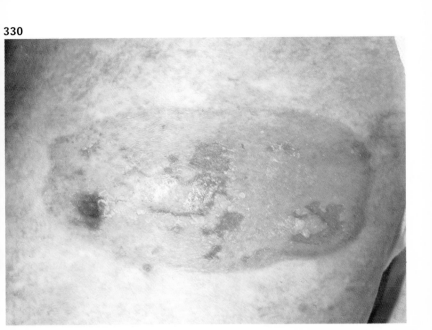

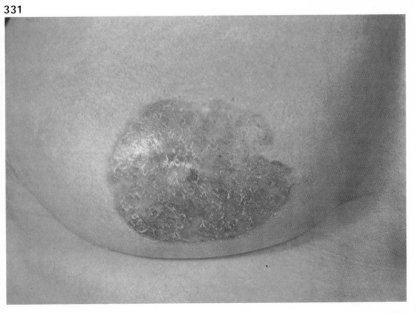

332 *Kaposi's sarcoma (multiple idiopathic haemorrhagic sarcoma), legs* Purple or brownish plaques and nodules appear on the feet and legs (occasionally elsewhere). It may at first resemble stasis purpura. Histological examination of a skin biopsy is necessary to confirm the diagnosis. Lesions progress very slowly.

333 *Metastasis, carcinomatous, cheek* This lesion had grown rapidly. Histology showed an undifferentiated carcinoma. The scalp is also a common site for metastases.

334 *Metastases, Hodgkin's disease, back* Large purple lesions with ulceration are seen. Lymphosarcoma may produce very similar lesions.

335 *Metastases, thigh* Pink nodules of lymphosarcoma. Metastases often first appear as small skin-coloured or pale pink nodules, and biopsy is necessary to prove the diagnosis and to classify the tumour.

332

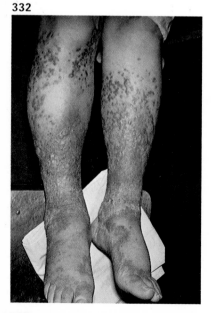

333

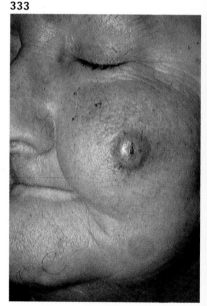

334

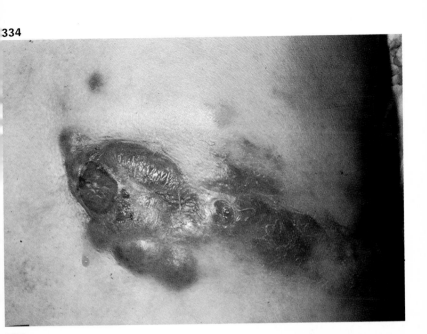

335

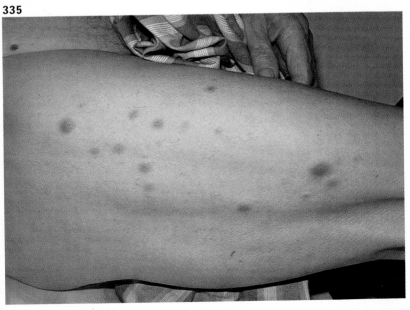

URTICARIAS AND ERYTHEMAS

By *urticaria* is meant the development of transient pruritic weals. Individual lesions may be papules, arcs or plaques and they rarely last longer than 12 hours. Histologically there is dermal oedema and vasodilatation with minimal cellular infiltrate.

The term *erythema* as applied to a disease state indicates the development of erythematous lesions which last for days, weeks or longer and are characterised histologically by dermal oedema, vasodilatation and the presence of a marked perivascular inflammatory cell infiltration.

336 *Urticaria, back* Irregular white or pink transient pruritic weals. This is the most common pattern. *Acute* urticaria may be provoked by an ingested food or drug or an acute infection. In *chronic* urticaria a cause is rarely found.

337 *Urticaria, figurate, back* Rapidly expanding annular or figurate lesions are often seen.

338 *Urticaria, cholinergic* Crops of small pruritic papules come with exertion and last for an hour or two. Usually found in adolescents and young adults, precipitated by heat, exercise or emotion.

336

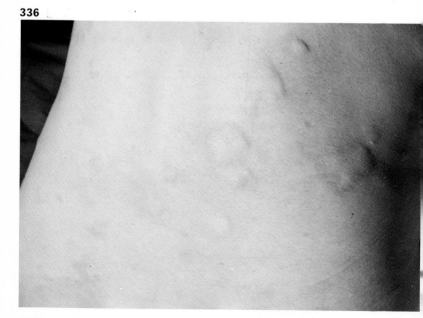

339 *Cold urticaria, ice test* In this condition weals arise on skin chilled by cold wind or water. Often, as here, application of ice for a minute or so will induce a weal but this response is variable.

340 *Dermographism, back* An exaggerated weal and flare reaction at sites of firm pressure with a blunt point. Lesions are also induced by scratching. It can occur in normal individuals.

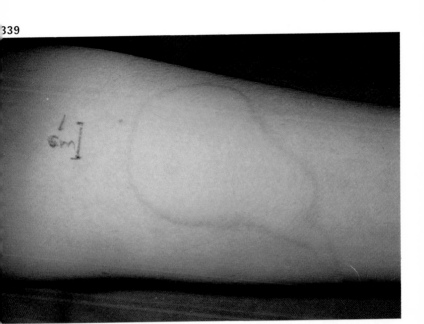

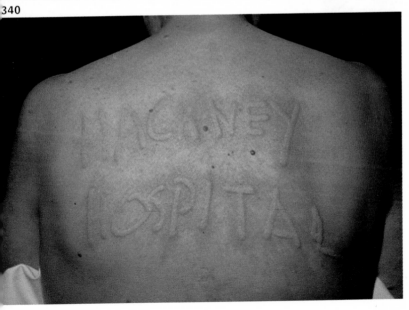

341 *Angio-oedema (angioneurotic oedema), face* This term indicates urticaria affecting the subcutaneous tissue, especially the face, tongue and larynx. The figure shows a mild form with swelling of the lip. In severe cases the face may be grossly swollen with the eyes closed by eyelid oedema and respiratory obstruction due to laryngeal oedema. It may be associated with acute and chronic urticaria. There is also a very rare familial type of angio-oedema in which deaths during attacks are recorded.

342 *'Toxic' erythema* A common clinical picture, of acute onset, with bright erythema of the extremities, elbows, knees and buttocks associated with pruritus. It may be associated with a bacterial or viral infection, drug ingestion, or malignant disease, but often no cause is found

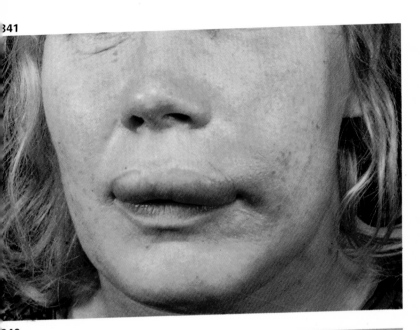

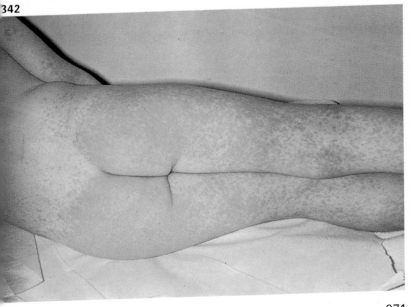

343 'Toxic' erythema, infectious mononucleosis This is a non-specific erythema. The buttocks were the site of maximum rash and some lesions were purpuric. Normally the incidence of skin rash in infectious mononucleosis is 5 – 10%. If ampicillin has been given at the sore throat stage, the incidence of rash approaches 100%.

344 'Toxic' erythema, probably drug induced This profuse eruption started about 10 days after beginning a course of oral penicillin. It is non-specific in appearance, and it may be impossible to be sure whether the eruption results from the drug, the underlying condition for which the drug was given, or from some other cause. If the same rash occurs when the patient is challenged with the drug at a later date, this is good evidence of a drug aetiology.

343

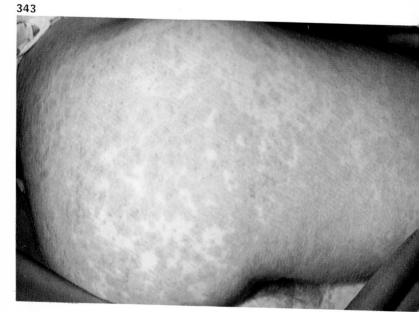

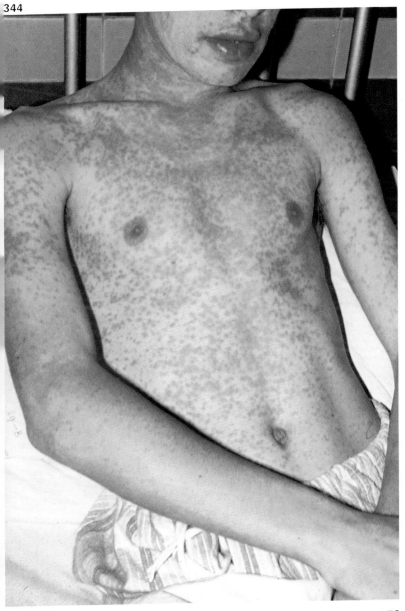

345 'Toxic' erythema, neck This eruption came on soon after a course of nifuratel tablets. The drug was later given again without a recurrence of the rash. The relationship between the drug and the rash is therefore in doubt and it is probably unjustified to label this as a 'drug eruption'.

346 Fixed drug eruption, bullous, hallux This lesion was provoked by a barbiturate.

347 Fixed drug eruption, dorsal hands There was an intense erythema with scaling and pruritus. It started a few hours after taking a single dose of salazosulphapyridine. The patient recalled having lesions in the same sites when he had taken the drug several years previously. It is a feature of this type of drug reaction that there is pruritic redness and swelling *at the same site* each time the drug is taken. Blisters may be produced. Post-inflammatory hyperpigmentation is common and can persist indefinitely. Drugs which are commonly responsible for fixed eruptions are sulphonamides, phenolphthalein and barbiturates.

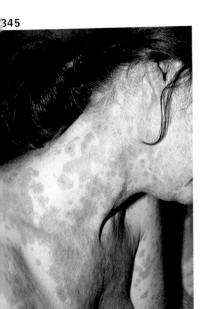

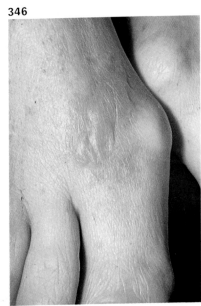

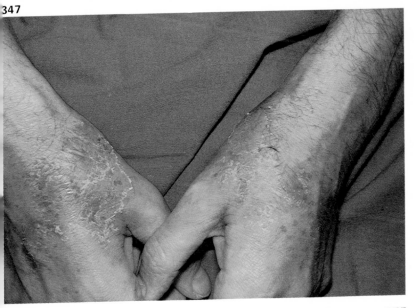

348 *Erythema multiforme, palms* This term should not be regarded as synonymous with 'toxic' erythemas, even annular ones. It is best reserved for a symmetrical eruption of iris-like ('target') lesions, with or without central blisters, affecting predominantly the hands and feet and spreading proximally to an extent depending on the severity. It comes on acutely, lasts 2–3 weeks and usually resolves spontaneously. It can be precipitated by herpes simplex, vaccination and drugs and may be recurrent. A similar condition but less well-defined may be associated with leukaemias and other reticuloses, carcinomas, and following x-ray therapy.

349 *Erythema multiforme* Close-up of palmar lesions. The concentric 'target' lesions are well shown, they are not as multiform as the label would suggest.

350 *Erythema multiforme, Stevens-Johnson syndrome* This syndrome consists of cutaneous erythema multiforme with ulceration of the mouth and often the eyes, nose and genital orifices as well. It can be very severe with high fever, prostration and a prolonged course. Systemic corticosteroids may be life-saving.

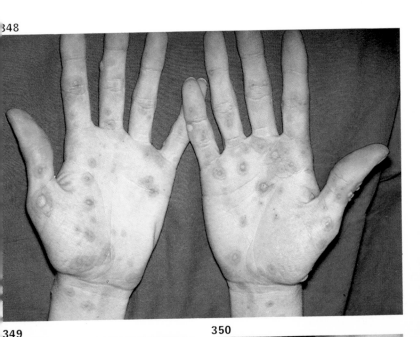

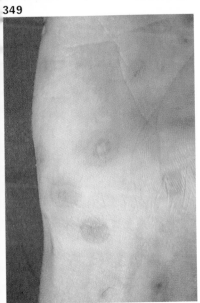

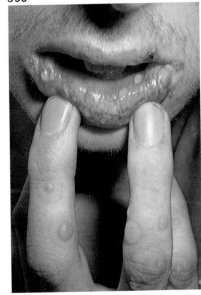

351 *Erythema nodosum* The characteristic site is the front of the shins. Early lesions are bright red, raised and tender. The common predisposing causes are acute sarcoidosis, streptococcal infections, drugs and primary tuberculosis, of which this skin eruption may be the presenting sign. Lesions may also occur on the thighs, arms and face, especially if a drug (e.g. sulphonamide) has been the cause.

352 *Erythema nodosum* Later stage, the lesions have flattened and have the appearance of resolving bruises.

353 *Erythema induratum (Bazin)* Tender deep dermal nodules develop in the calves. They may discharge but the contents are sterile. Scarring is a feature if discharge occurs. It is a sign of active tuberculosis although it is rarely possible to find the focus. In genuine cases the tuberculin reaction is strongly positive and antituberculous therapy is curative. However it must be stressed that non-tuberculous forms of recurrent leg nodules are found, especially in middle-aged women. The condition may be called erythema induratum (Whitfield), nodular vasculitis or panniculitis. A cause is rarely found.

354 *Erythema annulare centrifugum* The rings gradually spread outwards with central clearing. Skin biopsy may be necessary to be sure it is not a lymphoma. Usually no cause is found and the lesions eventually stop appearing after months or years.

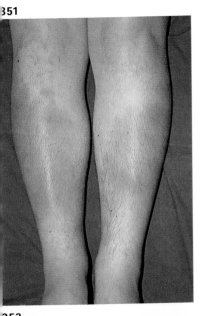

351

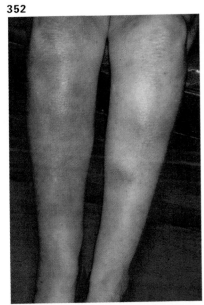

352

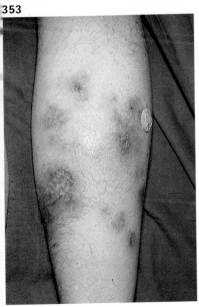

353

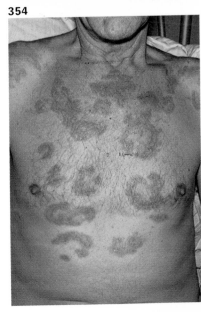

354

355 *Palmar erythema ('liver palms')* This condition only rarely denotes liver disease, being found in many chronic disorders such as pulmonary tuberculosis and rheumatoid arthritis, or even in normal people.

356 *Erythema ab igne* This pigmented and reticulate erythema is due to sitting with the legs too close to a fire over a long period in winter. In summer only pigmentation may remain. It appears on the surfaces of the shins closest to the heat so that usually only one side of each shin is involved. It must be distinguished from livedo reticularis (**450**) which can be associated with systemic disease.

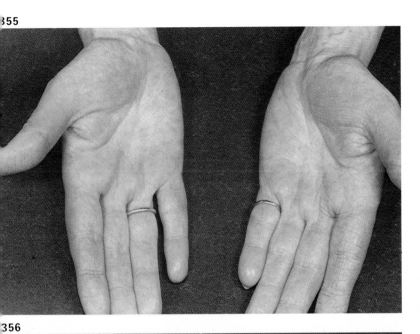

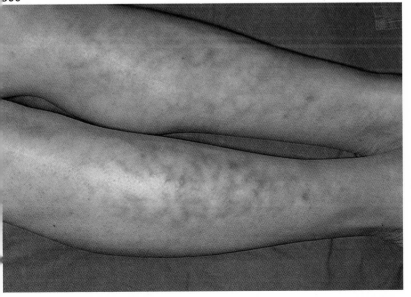

PURPURA, VASCULITIS AND OTHER VASCULAR DISORDERS

In this group of disorders pathological changes are seen histologically in or around the vessels. It should be remembered that vascular damage can occur as an end-result of a variety of mechanisms (e.g. traumatic, infective, biochemical, immunological).

357 *Purpura, axilla, due to scratching* The trauma of scratching has damaged capillaries without breaking the skin. The purpura is incidental.

358 *Purpura, 'senile' type, dorsal hand and wrist* Purpura on trivial trauma is common on areas of skin with a thinned dermis due to old age and previous sun exposure, or systemic corticosteroid therapy. Lesions are slow to resolve.

359 *Purpura, clothing, chest* Pressure from clothing with an open texture may produce purpura, especially in children. It does not indicate an underlying systemic disorder.

357

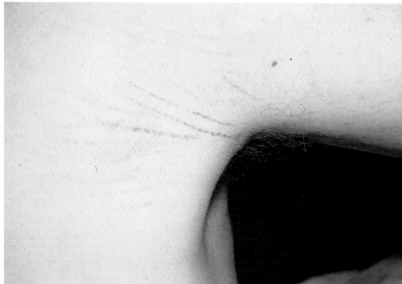

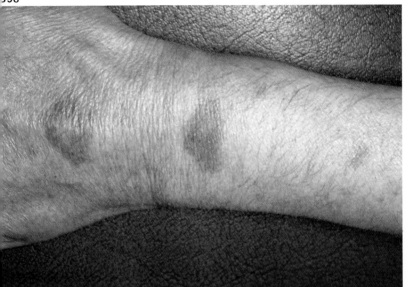

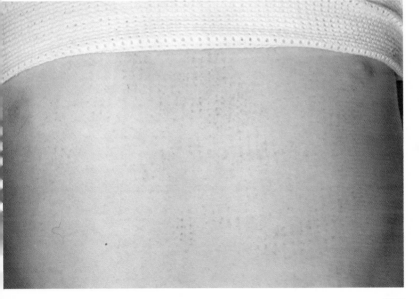

360 *White atrophy (atrophie blanche), leg and ankle* White depressed irregular areas of scarring often found in association with stasis purpura or healed ulcers. Secondary painful ulceration may follow.

361 *Purpura, stasis, leg and ankle* Often associated with varicose veins. The brownish colour is characteristic. Gravitational ('varicose') eczema and ulceration may be associated.

362 *Purpura, thrombocytopenic, thigh and leg* Spontaneous bleeding into normal skin is seen. The patient had aplastic anaemia. Trauma may result in large bruises (ecchymoses).

360

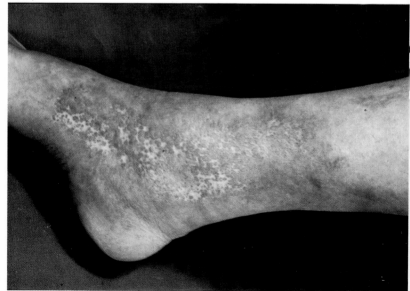

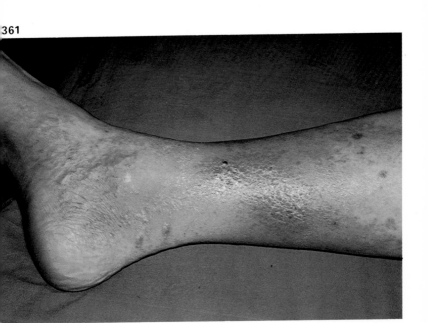

361

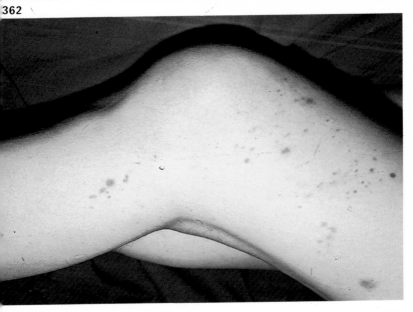

362

287

363 *Purpura, uraemic, back* Occasionally a presenting sign of chronic renal failure.

364 *Chilblains (perniosis), foot* Red itchy oedematous lesions (cold to the touch) appear on extremities a few hours after exposure to cold, and take several days to resolve. They are common in children and young adults.

365 *Purpura, cutaneous vasculitis, legs* There is damage to superficial blood vessels with small infarcts of the skin. Purpura is invariable and is associated with necrotic blisters, and ulcers. Lesions come usually in crops, which may be recurrent, mostly on the legs and feet. Acute vasculitis associated with gut, renal joint and other lesions is called 'Henoch-Schönlein Purpura'. Infections and drugs are often suspected of causing cutaneous vasculitis but it is difficult to prove this.

363

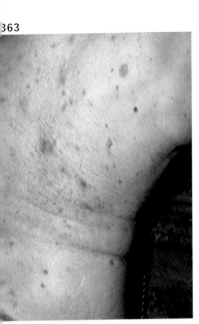

364

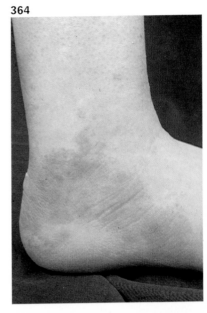

365

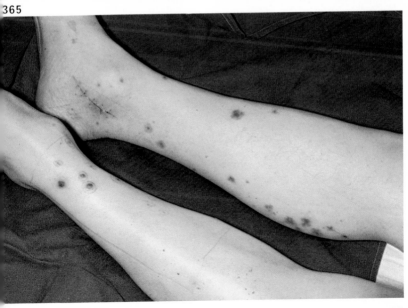

366 *Purpura, cutaneous vasculitis, ankle* Irregular purpuric infarcts with blisters and epidermal necrosis are seen.

367 *Pigmented purpuric eruption, legs* A chronic eruption of discrete or confluent reddish-brown spots (like cayenne pepper) with some epidermal thickening and scaling, usually confined to the feet and legs. Some cases are a drug reaction from taking carbromal or meprobamate. These clear when the drug is stopped. In many cases no cause is found. Histology shows a capillaritis.

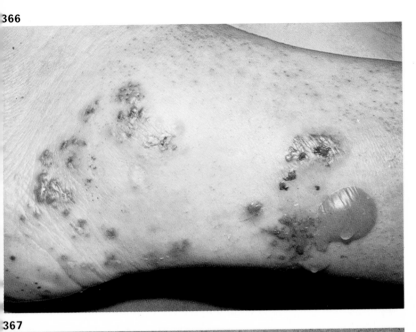

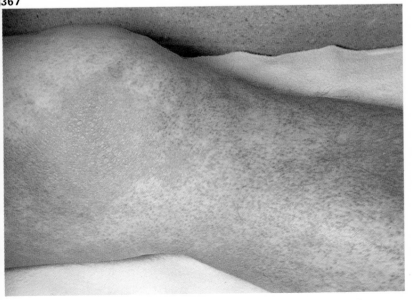

368 *Behçet's syndrome, tongue* There were several painful ulcers in the posterior mouth and pharynx. They were recurrent, both in the mouth and on the uvula, for several years. In this patient the uvula had been destroyed by repeated ulceration.

369 *Behçet's syndrome, scrotum* A group of deep painful ulcers on the scrotum.

370 *Behçet's syndrome, vulva* Recurrent oro-genital ulceration is part of this disorder. The ulcers show no specific features clinically or histologically.

371 *Gangrene, toes* This was the result of atheroma of the large arteries of the legs. It is sometimes seen as a complication of diabetes.

368

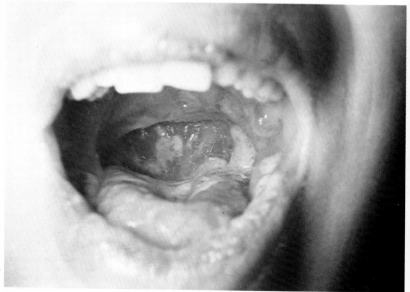

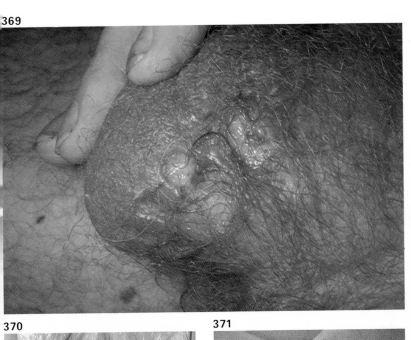

369

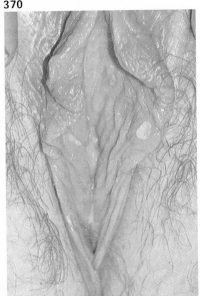

370

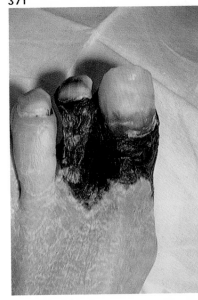

371

372 *Varicose ulcers, lower legs* These ulcers are common in elderly women with varicose veins and stasis purpura. They are confined to the lower legs and are often complicated by infection and allergic contact dermatitis to topical medicaments. Bacteriological examination of swabs for pathogens is necessary to detect infection, and patch testing often reveals unsuspected allergic contact dermatitis.

373 *Leg ulcers, in sickle-cell anaemia* It must be remembered that not all leg ulcers are 'varicose' ulcers. This figure shows ulcers associated with sickle-cell anaemia. Other possible causes include trauma, hypertension, late syphilis, rheumatoid arthritis, diabetes, spherocytosis, arterio-venous aneurysms and malignant tumours. In general, venous ulcers are large and painless and around the ankle whereas arterial ulcers are small, painful and on the shin or side of the leg.

374 *Chondrodermatitis nodularis helicis* There is a hyperkeratotic nodule on the rim of the helix. These lesions occur mostly in elderly men and they can be very painful. Trauma, poor blood supply and probably light exposure play a part in their production. There is frequently secondary involvement of the underlying cartilage.

372

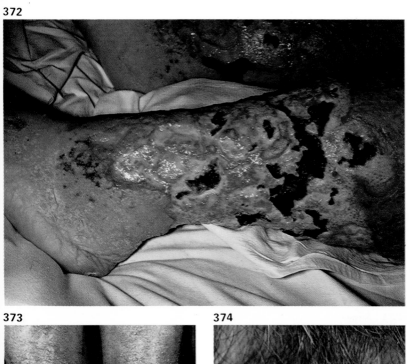

373

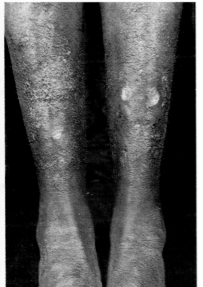

374

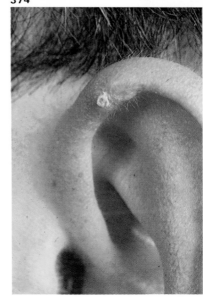

375 *Arborescent telangiectasia, leg* Leashes of dilated superficial veins are seen. Minor degrees are very common in middle age.

376 *Haemangioma, cavernous* The 'strawberry naevus' starts in the first few weeks of life and grows for many months. It can be expected to resolve spontaneously without cosmetic defect by the age of 10.

377 *Haemangioma, capillary* The 'port-wine stain' is present at birth and is permanent. On the head it may be associated with a meningeal haemangioma, a rare cause of epilepsy.

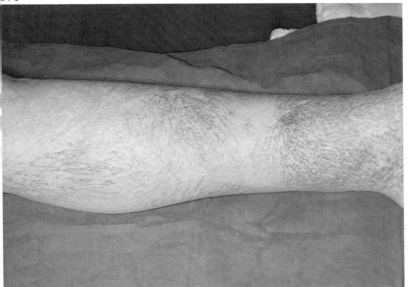

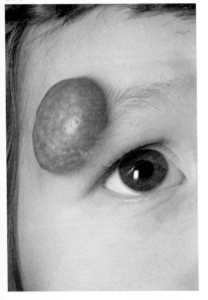

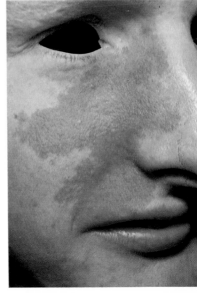

378 *Spider naevus, cheek* A central bright red spot is surrounded by radiating red 'legs'. The central spot is a dilated arteriole. It can be temporarily obliterated by central pressure on the lesion with a fine pointed instrument, but refills at once when the pressure is removed. Single lesions are commonly found on the face, trunk and limbs in healthy children and adults and they may enlarge during pregnancy. Numerous lesions may be found in association with hepatic cirrhosis.

379 *Naevus anaemicus, thigh* This presents as a circumscribed patch of pale skin of normal texture. It is due mainly to increased sensitivity of the vessels to catecholamines. They are usually seen on the trunk.

380 *Venous lake, lip* A soft compressible dark blue blood-filled papule found on the lips in the elderly.

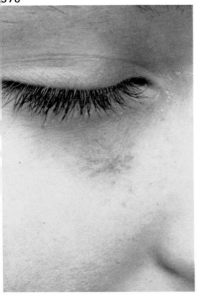

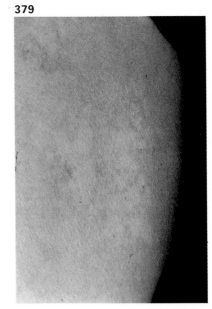

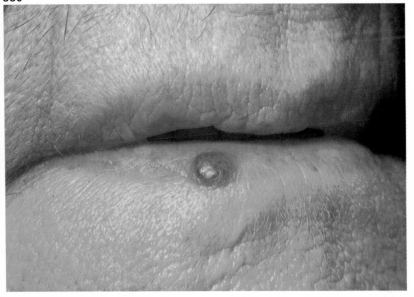

381 *'Senile' haemangiomata (cherry angiomas, Campbell de Morgan spots), abdomen* Very common from middle life onwards these small bright red papules are found mostly on the front of the chest and abdomen. They cannot be emptied with pressure.

382 *Angiokeratomas of scrotum* Numerous small dark red papules are seen on the scrotal skin. They are due to grossly dilated dermal vessels, usually with overlying hyperkeratosis. In the common Fordyce type they increase with advancing age and are of no special significance. Rarely, they are part of angiokeratoma corporis diffusum (Anderson-Fabry disease), a sex-linked disorder of sphingolipid metabolism characterised clinically by multiple angiokeratomas in the bathing-drawers area, intermittent pain in fingers and toes from childhood onwards and progressive renal damage detectable in the third decade of life.

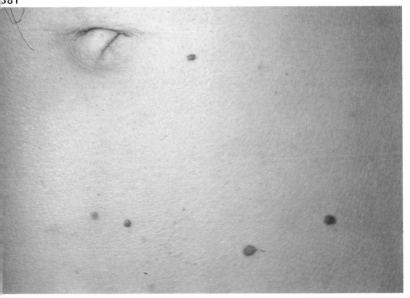

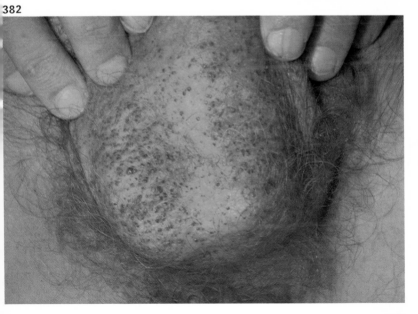

383 Lymphoedema, hereditary (Milroy's disease) Lifelong symptomless non-pitting oedema is present. It can be unilateral or bilateral, and is due to a congenital defect of the lymphatic vessels. Impaired lymphatic spread of injected dye is shown in the more oedematous left leg.

384 Glomus tumour, wrist In this case a small very tender purple papule was present on the outer aspect of the wrist. The extremities are the favoured sites and lesions under the nail plate are particularly painful. Multiple tumours, often painless, are seen in children. Excision cures.

385 Lymphangioma Clusters of small deep vesicles are seen. Haemorrhage into the lesions is common. They are often far more extensive than their superficial appearance indicates.

383

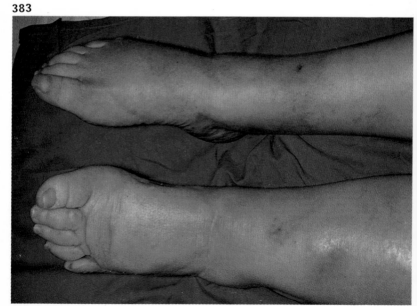

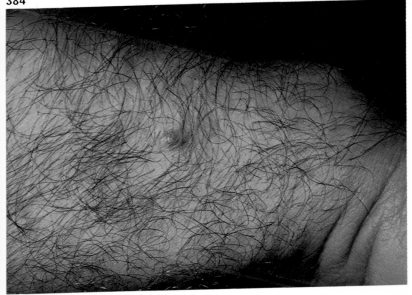

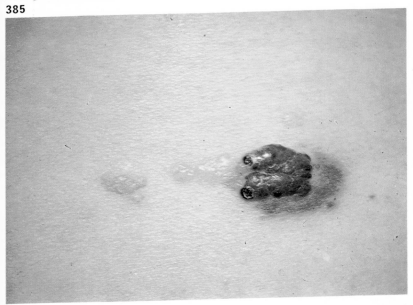

386 *Lupus erythematosus, face* Typical chronic lesions show redness, scaling, telangiectasia, atrophy, and variable pigmentary changes.

387 *Lupus erythematosus, face* Lesions of recent onset are symmetrical, red and oedematous. They are often most pronounced on the areas of the face which receive most light exposure ; i.e. the upper cheeks and bridge of the nose, and the prominences of the forehead. Acute systemic lupus erythematosus of the face may resemble sunburn erythema.

388 *Lupus erythematosus, ear* The ear lobes and adjacent areas are frequently affected.

389 *Lupus erythematosus, scalp* Red plaque with loss of hair, which is often permanent, producing a scarring alopecia.

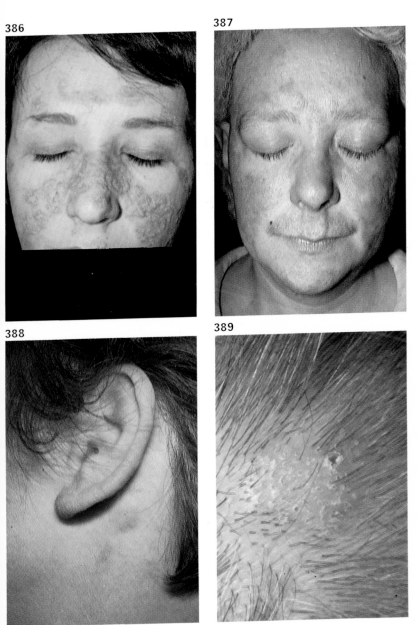

386

387

388

389

390 *Lupus erythematosus, fingers* Lesions on the dorsa of the proximal phalanges are characteristic.

391 *Lupus erythematosus, fingers* Chronic lesions of fingers and toes may show hyperkeratosis and variable atrophy.

392 *Lupus erythematosus, vasculitis, toes* Small purpuric macules are seen.

390

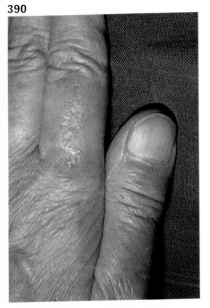

391

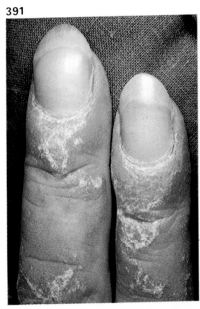

392

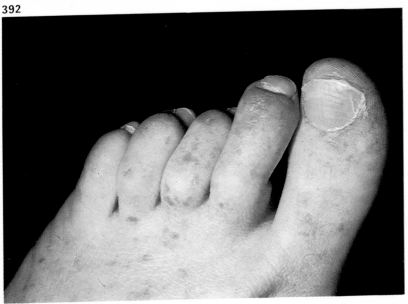

393 *Localised scleroderma (morphoea), trunk* Oedematous plaques with a mauve edge and central induration. At a later stage the discoloration may fade.

394 *Localised scleroderma, back* This extensive lesion had been present for many years.

395 *Scleroderma, face* Tight skin over the forehead, cheeks and nose gives the face a 'pinched' appearance. In severe cases the oral aperture may be reduced in size, making insertion and removal of dentures difficult.

396 *Scleroderma, face* Macular telangiectases are common in systemic scleroderma. They are more than usually profuse in this patient.

393

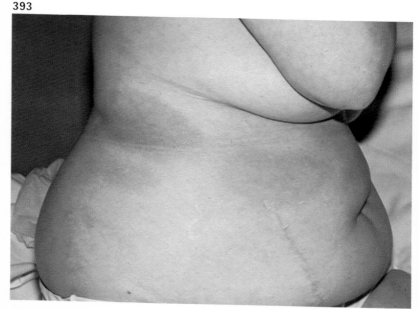

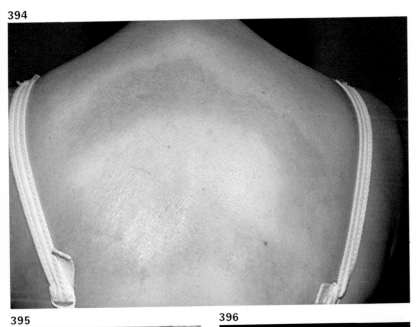

394

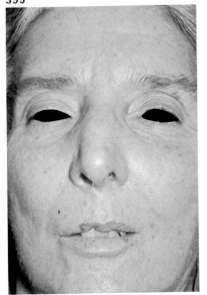

395

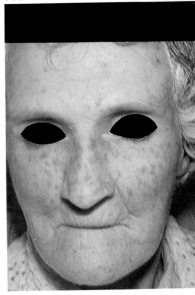

396

397 *Systemic sclerosis, hands* Indurated shiny hyperpigmented hands with flexion deformity of the fingers is seen in some advanced cases.

398 *Systemic sclerosis, hand with ischaemic ulcers* Chronic painful ulcers over the dorsal finger joints. Calcinosis may be present and will be demonstrated readily by x-rays of the hands.

399 *Dermatomyositis, face, trunk and arm* The bright magenta ('heliotrope') colour is characteristic. In this patient the disease was associated with breast cancer. Malignant disease is present in about a quarter of adult cases.

400 *Dermatomyositis, face* The symmetrical magenta colour with oedema, affecting particularly the upper eyelids is virtually patho-gnomonic.

397

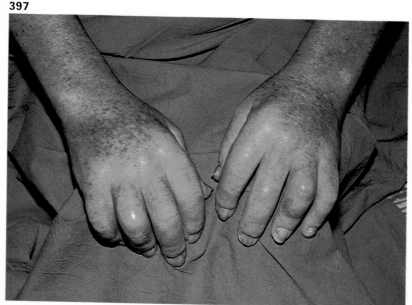

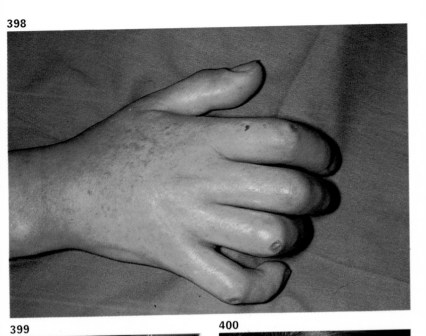

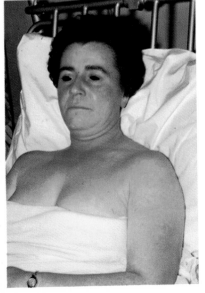

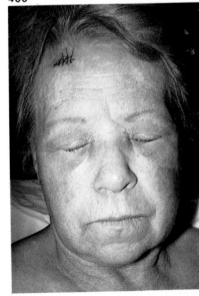

401 *Dermatomyositis, nape of neck* The magenta colour is superimposed on a weather-beaten neck. The patient had lung cancer.

402 *Dermatomyositis, chest, Negro* The pattern and symmetrical distribution is typical of dermatomyositis but, as often happens in negroid skin, erythema is partially obscured by inflammatory hyperpigmentation.

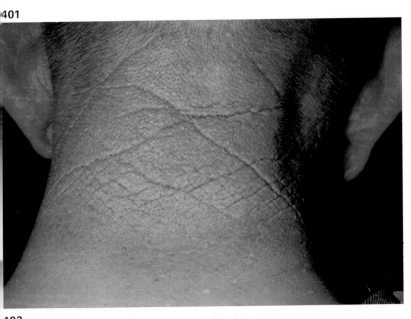

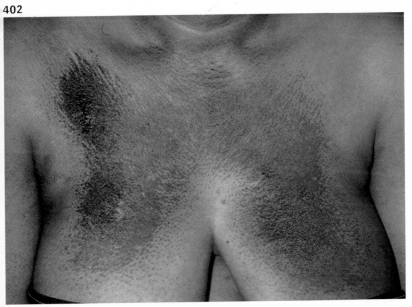

403 *Dermatomyositis, dorsal hands* There is erythema over the dorsal metacarpel-phalangeal joints and the proximal interphalangeal joints. There is also a tendency for the erythema to be streaked along the extensor tendons. This pattern is characteristic of dermatomyositis and is to be distinguished from that of lupus erythematosus (see **390**) where the erythema is over the dorsal proximal phalanx with sparing of the knuckles.

404 *Dermatomyositis, nail fold telangiectasia* Nail fold telangiectasia with vascular thromboses, scarring and ragged cuticles is particularly characteristic of dermatomyositis. It is also found, often less extremely, in scleroderma and in systemic lupus erythematosus.

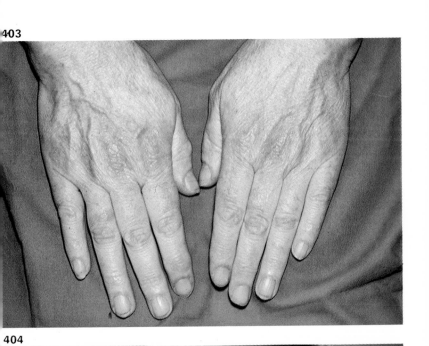

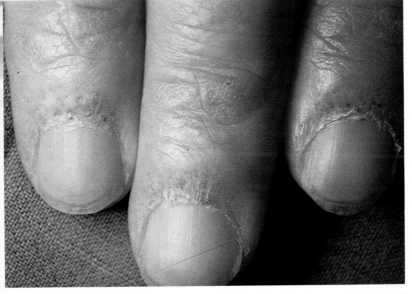

405 *Dermatomyositis, scarring alopecia* Chronic dermatomyositis in young people can produce considerable scarring.

406 *Dermatomyositis, calcinosis cutis* Calcinotic nodules, especially around joints, may be a prominent feature of the disease in young people. Similar lesions are seen in systemic sclerosis.

407 *Polyarteritis nodosa, ankle and foot* Livedo reticularis with chronic painful ulceration is sometimes seen in this disease.

405

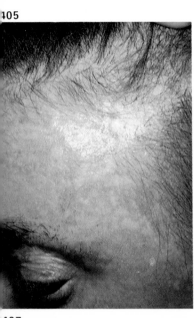

406

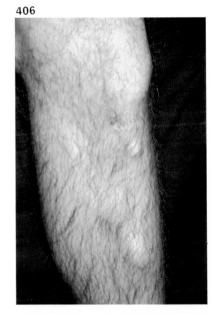

407

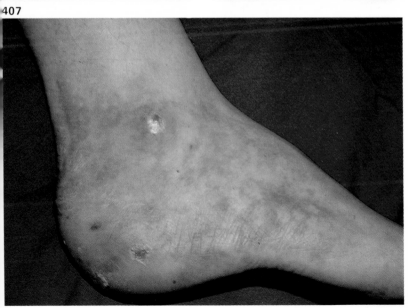

LIGHT-INDUCED DERMATOSES

Daylight and sunlight cause slow but progressive damage to the skin. The familiar skin changes of old age (i.e. atrophy, wrinkling, telangiectasia, pigmentary anomalies and elastosis) are seen predominantly on the areas exposed to ultra-violet irradiation (the face, neck and dorsal hands). Sunlight exposure is an important aetiological factor in the production of many skin tumours (e.g. solar keratoses, **312**; keratoacanthomas, **309, 310**; basal cell carcinomas, **320–322**; squamous carcinomas, **325, 326**; and facial malignant melanomas, **318**).

A patient is said to be 'light-sensitive' when his skin reacts pathologically, within hours or days, to a degree of light exposure which would not normally induce more than a mild erythema. The abnormal response may be papular, erythematous, eczematous or bullous.

408 *Light-induced telangiectasia of neck ('chicken neck')* This disorder is seen usually in fair-skinned, middle-aged women who have had excessive light exposure.

409 *Solar elastosis, nose* There are yellowish small plaques of thickened skin on the nose. They occur in elderly, fair-skinned individuals and are a consequence of prolonged sunlight exposure. Similar lesions are found on the prominences of the forehead and at the back of the neck. This man also has comedones (blackheads) around the eyes, a frequent associated feature.

410 *Polymorphic light eruption, face* The primary feature is the production of itchy papules, instead of normal sunburn erythema, by sunlight. They come up a few hours after significant sun exposure during the summer months and last a few days. The changes seen are those of dermatitis/eczema.

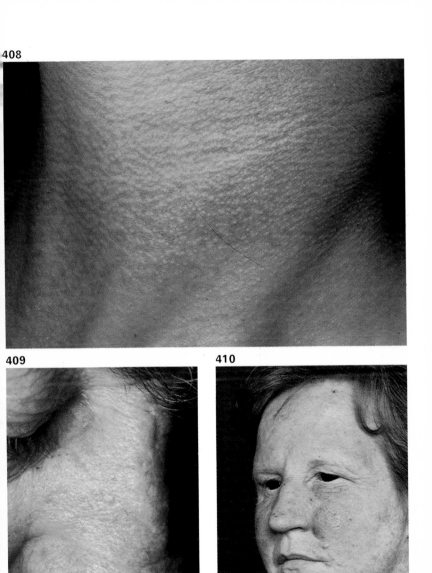

411 *Light eruption, face and neck* An intense inflammation of light-exposed areas. Possible causes are ingested drugs (especially tranquillizers and sulphonamides) and topical photosensitising applications.

412 *Porphyria cutanea tarda, face* Scarring and pigmentary changes are present. Hypertrichosis is also common. Suffused eyelids and conjunctivae are frequently seen.

413 *Porphyria cutanea tarda, chest* There is induration and hyperpigmentation with surrounding erythema, giving an appearance similar to scleroderma.

414 *Porphyria cutanea tarda, hand* There is often a history of increased skin fragility. Sometimes the only clinical sign of porphyria is the presence of brownish ill-defined macules with minimal atrophy on the backs of the hands. The brown marks are healed erosions or ulcers, produced by minor trauma. Similar lesions are seen in porphyria variegata. The patient may deny aggravation of lesions by exposure to sunlight.

411

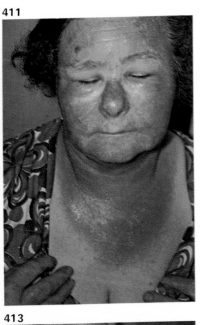

412

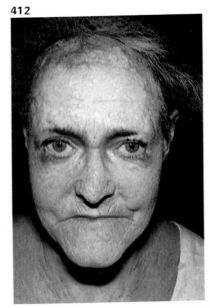

413

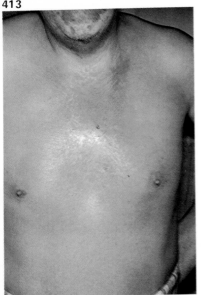

414

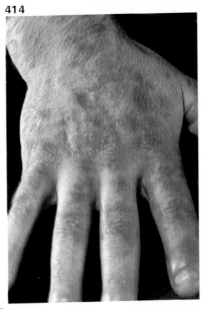

415 *Porphyria cutanea tarda, dorsal hands* There is mottled hyper and hypo-pigmentation with scarring and erosions on the light-exposed areas of the dorsal hands and forearms.

416 *Porphyria cutanea tarda, dorsal hand with blisters* Blisters may be small and easily overlooked, but they often leave scars studded with milia (see **285**).

415

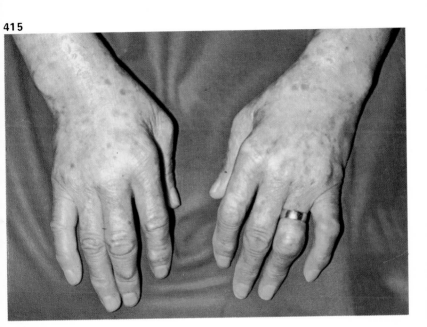

416

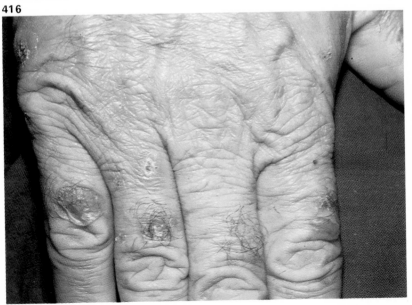

417 *Actinic reticuloid, back of neck* The sharp line around the neck where the collar protects the skin from the effects of light is particularly characteristic of a light-induced dermatosis.

418 *Actinic reticuloid, face* A confluent red oedematous dermatitis of light-exposed areas. It tends to occur in older men with a pre-existing dermatitis/eczema. The name 'reticuloid' refers to the histology which may give an impression of a reticulosis.

419 *Erythropoietic protoporphyria, nose scars* Light sensitivity starts in infancy or early childhood. Scars on the nose are commonly found but are not always conspicuous.

420 *Erythropoietic protoporphyria, dorsal hand scars* Skin changes in this disease may be very subtle. Thickening is seen and felt over the dorsum of the index metacarpo-phalangeal joint.

417

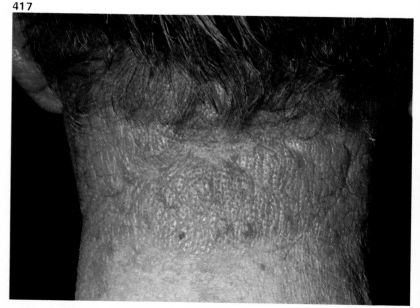

418

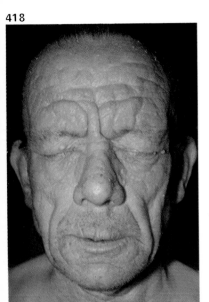

419

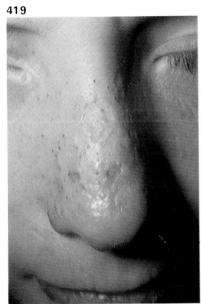

420

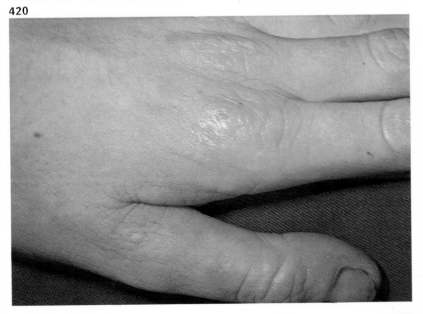

421 *Xeroderma pigmentosum, face* A mild example. There is profuse rather irregular freckling with mild atrophic changes over the nose.

422 *Xeroderma pigmentosum, face* A more severe case than **421**. Freckling on light-exposed areas is grosser and atrophic changes are seen on the nose, cheeks and lips. Keratoses, basal cell and squamous carcinomas and melanomas arise on the damaged skin.

423 *Hutchinson's summer prurigo* A distinctive dermatosis. The patient is a child with excoriated eczematous lesions on light-exposed areas. It may be mistakenly diagnosed as atopic dermatitis.

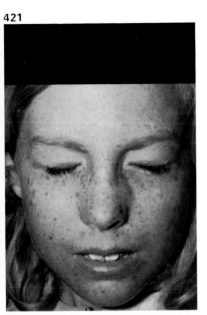

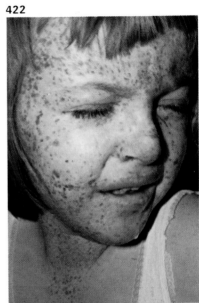

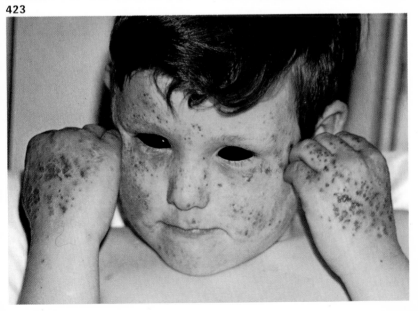

SKIN MANIFESTATIONS OF SYSTEMIC DISEASE

424 *Sarcoidosis, in scars* Brownish papules have appeared in old scars on the front of the knee. Sites of scarring should always be inspected if sarcoidosis is in question.

425 *Sarcoidosis, in tribal markings, chest*

426 *Sarcoidosis, eyelid* Plaques of sarcoidosis are seen at the inner canthus and on the upper eyelid.

424

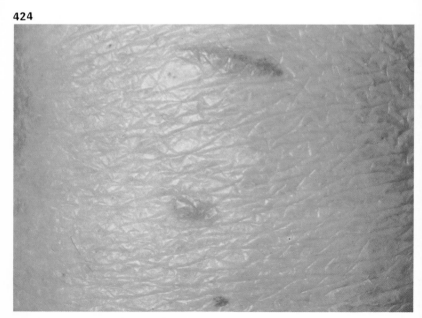

425

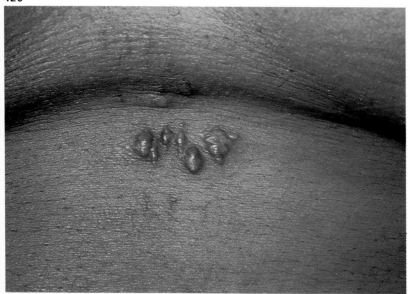

426

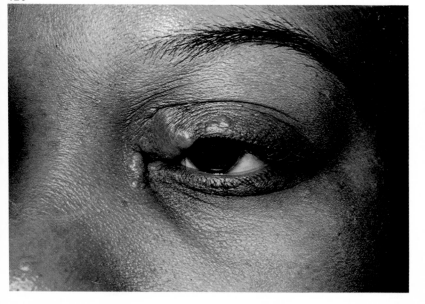

427 *Sarcoidosis, nose* The skin around the nostrils is distended by sarcoid tissue. A similar appearance may be seen in lupus vulgaris and leprosy.

428 *Sarcoidosis, nose, (lupus pernio)* The bluish-red shiny tip of the nose is characteristic.

429 *Sarcoidosis, plaques, legs*

430 *Sarcoidosis, back* Occasionally lesions are extensive and appear in annular form.

427

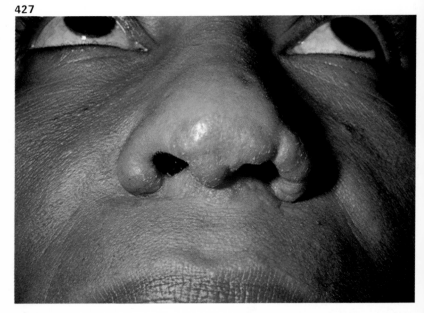

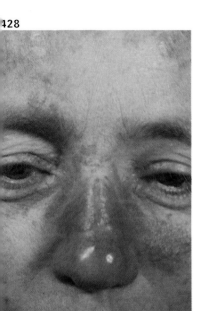

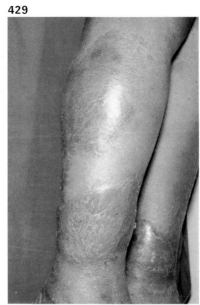

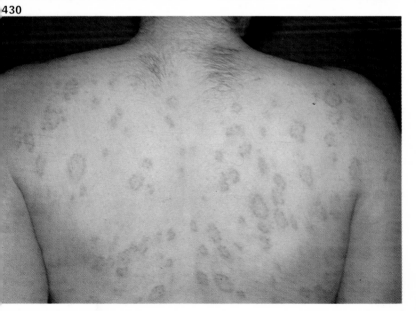

431 *Sarcoidosis, micropapular* Numerous lesions are seen around the nose. This form of sarcoidosis is common in American Negroes.

432 *Tuberous xanthomas, elbows* Pink or yellowish nodules on pressure areas. Regularly associated with blood lipid abnormalities.

433 *Tuberous xanthomas, knees* The nodules are pink rather than yellow.

431

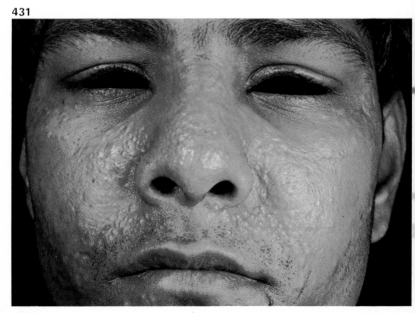

432

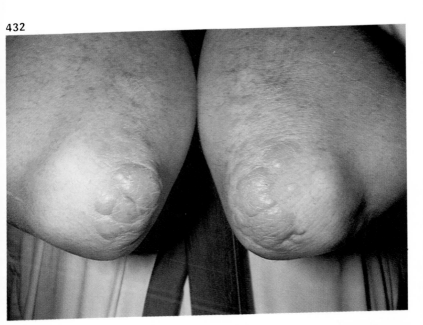

433

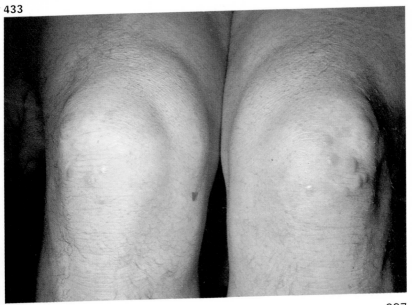

434 *Xanthelasmata* Yellow flat xanthomas affecting the inner aspects of the eyelids. It is only rarely that they are associated with blood lipid abnormalities.

435 *Eruptive xanthomas, back* A sudden eruption of profuse xanthomas may occur in liver disease with jaundice, lipoid nephrosis, diabetes mellitus, myxoedema and chronic pancreatitis.

434

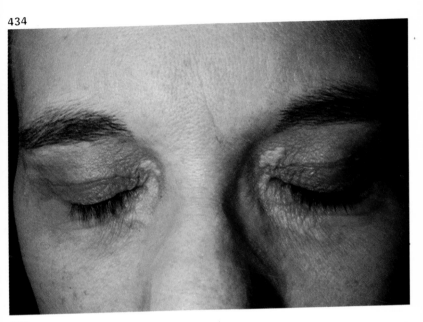

435

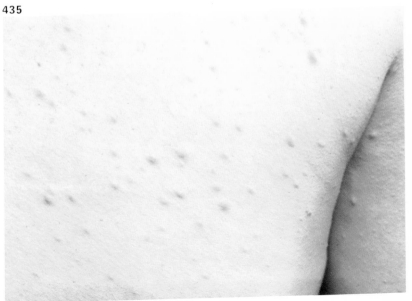

436 *Pseudoxanthoma elasticum, neck* Whitish or yellowish irregular plaques, streaks or papules in flexures, especially the sides of the neck and axillae. Involved skin is soft and lax. Associated with retinopathy ('angioid streaks'), arterial disease and gastrointestinal haemorrhage.

437 *Amyloidosis, tongue* The tongue is enlarged and is covered with translucent papules, many of which are haemorrhagic.

438 *Amyloidosis, lip* Waxy papules with purpura are characteristic.

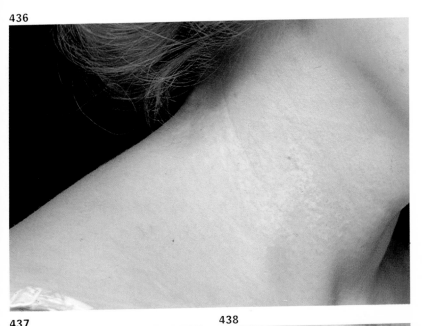

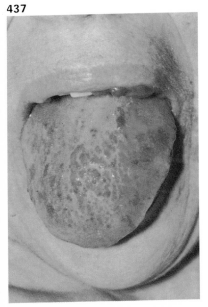

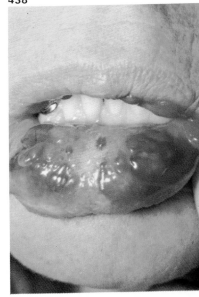

439 *Pretibial myxoedema, early* There are red oedematous swellings just above the lateral malleoli.

440 *Pretibial myxoedema, late* There is gross thickened oedema and erythema of the legs and feet. It usually follows surgical, chemical or isotope therapy for thyrotoxicosis.

441 *Necrobiosis lipoidica, shins* The skin lesions are sharply marginated, yellow or brownish-yellow areas of shiny atrophy with telangiectasia. Many but not all cases are diabetic.

439

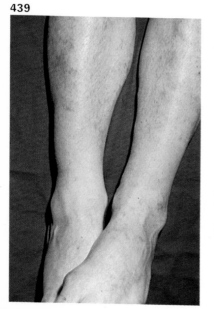

440

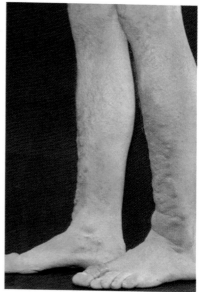

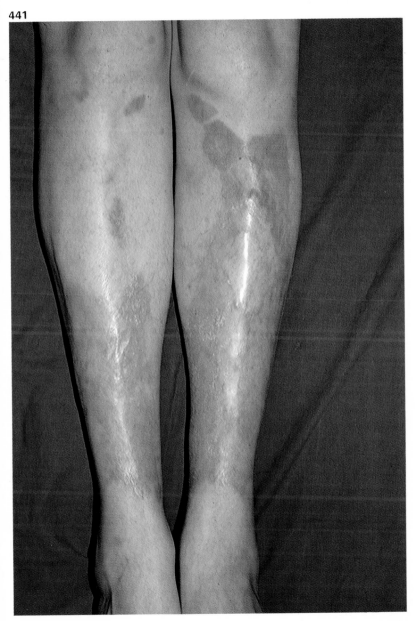

442 *Pyoderma gangrenosum, thigh* There is an advancing crusted edge with irregular exudative ulceration and central healing with scarring. These lesions may be associated with ulcerative colitis, arthritis, or a monoclonal gammopathy.

443 *Pyoderma gangrenosum, calf* A more active lesion than in **442** with marked inflammation and ulceration.

444 *'Toxic' erythema associated with Hodgkin's disease*
Lesions were widespread and pruritic ; a non-specific cutaneous association of malignant disease.

442

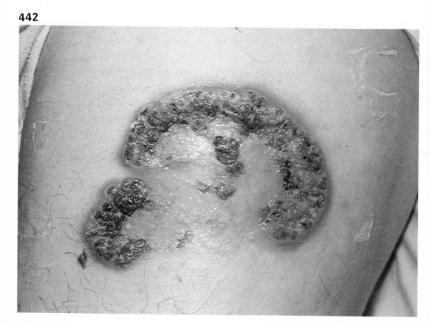

443

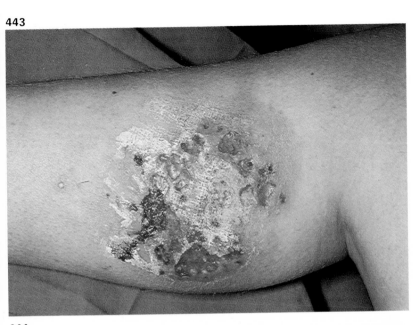

444

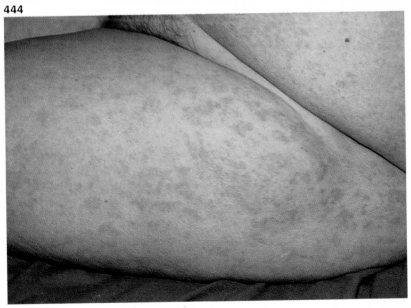

445 *Excoriations, Hodgkin's disease, shoulder* Lesions arise when the patient scratches a pruritic but normal looking skin. No malignant cells are found in histology of these lesions.

446 *Excoriations, uraemic, back* In this patient generalised pruritus was the presenting symptom of chronic renal failure. Scratch marks on hyperpigmented but otherwise normal skin are seen.

447 *Excoriations, obstructive jaundice, chest* Pruritus may be severe when jaundice is minimal. The patient should be examined in daylight, rather than artificial light, to detect mild jaundice clinically.

448 *Carotenaemia, palm* The patient's yellow palm (right) is compared with a normal palm. In an attempt to lose weight the patient was eating 1 kg raw carrots daily. The pigmentation resolved when she stopped eating carrots. The sclerae were unaffected. Mild forms sometimes occur in hypothyroidism, diabetes and hyperlipidaemia.

445

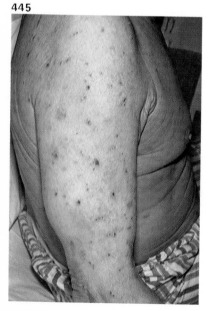

446

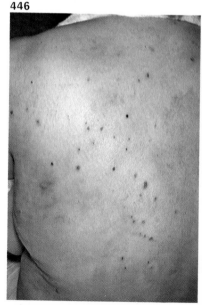

447

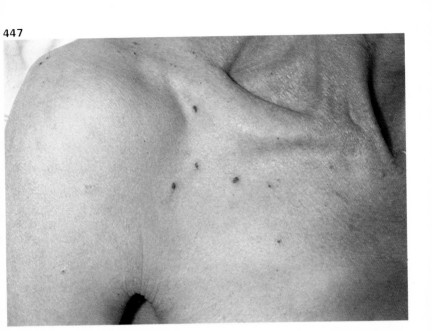

448

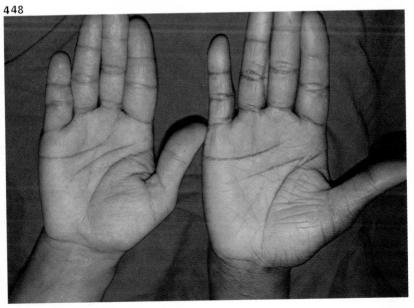

449 *Erythroderma, due to reticulosis* A generalised dry pruritic erythroderma may be associated with Hodgkin's disease or other reticulosis.

450 *Livedo reticularis, thighs* The appearance can be associated with peripheral vascular disease and with debilitating systemic diseases. This patient had bronchial carcinoma.

451 *Hereditary haemorrhagic telangiectasia (Osler-Rendu-Weber disease)* Multiple red spots on skin and mucous membranes. Epistaxis is common and there is usually a known family history of the condition.

449

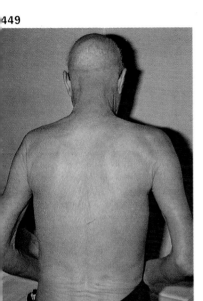

450

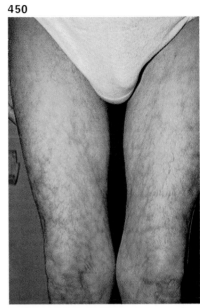

451

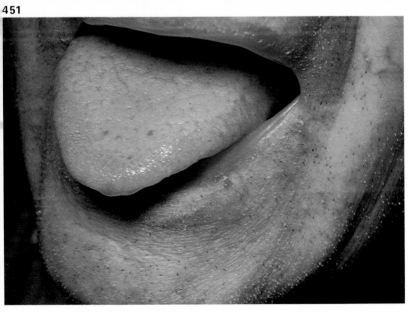

452 *Degos' disease (malignant atrophic papulosis), flexor aspect of wrist* A very rare disorder diagnosed by small round or oval pink papules with a depressed porcelain-white centre. Many cases terminate with lesions in the gut resulting in multiple perforations and fatal peritonitis.

453 *Acanthosis nigricans, perineum* Velvety rough thickening of flexural skin with increased pigmentation. Numerous scattered small warty lesions are also found. In adults this condition is regularly associated with malignant disease. A benign juvenile form also exists.

452

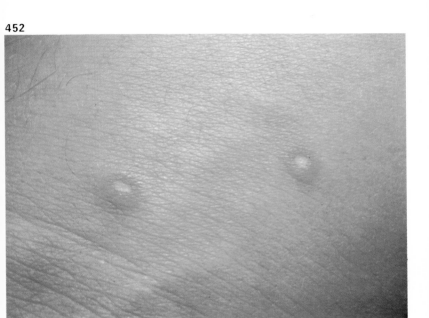

453

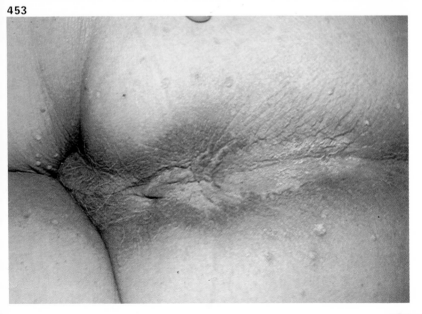

SELF-INDUCED DERMATOSES

Self-induced skin lesions may be the external manifestation of a wide variety of psychological disturbances. A high index of suspicion is often required to make the diagnosis. Lesions tend to be of bizarre shape or distribution which do not correspond to any familiar organic disease pattern. The production of lesions may be more or less unconscious and the patient will rarely confess that they are self-induced. In young people there is frequently a clear history of a disturbed family background and the prognosis is usually good. In middle-aged and elderly patients it may be extremely difficult to find the underlying psychological cause of the condition which tends to be extremely resistant to any form of treatment.

GRANULOMA ANNULARE & ATROPHIC DISORDERS

454 *Acne excoriée, cheek* The patient, a young woman, has scratched out real or imagined blemishes and small white scars remain. It can be regarded as a compulsive picking neurosis.

455 *Dermatitis artefacta, lips* The patient used a manicure set to produce these lesions.

456 *Dermatitis artefacta, side of face* New lesions were produced continually over many years and considerable scarring has resulted.

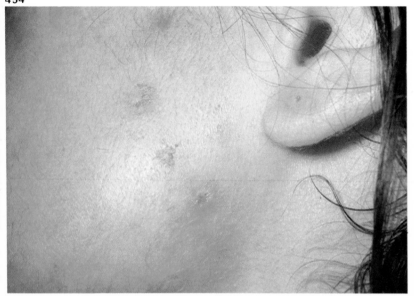

454

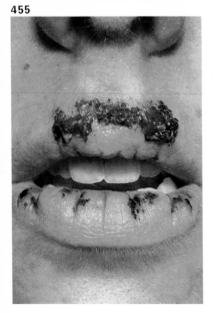

455

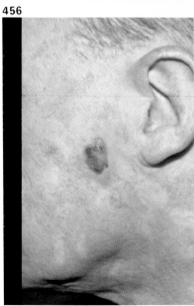

456

457 *Dermatitis artefacta, arms* These lesions were produced by a caustic fluid.

458 *Injection marks, elbow flexure* The patient was a young male drug addict.

457

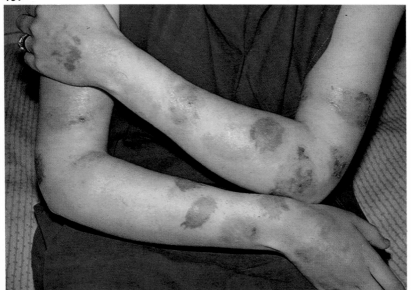

458

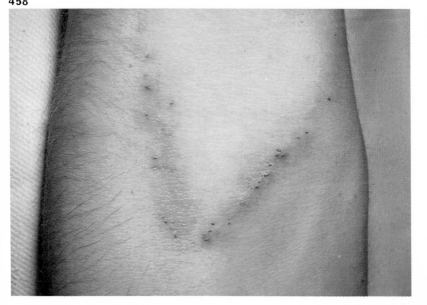

459 *Granuloma annulare, thumb* Lesions start as a nodule and slowly progress to a spreading ring. Histologically a dermal necrobiosis of collagen is seen. The exterior surfaces of the hand and fingers are common sites for granuloma annulare. Lesions tend to be more severe in diabetics.

460 *Granuloma annulare, dorsal foot* This is also a common site for the disease. The patient was a child and the lesion had been mis-diagnosed as ringworm. The hard raised edge and absence of scaling and pruritus are usually sufficient to distinguish it from a fungal infection.

459

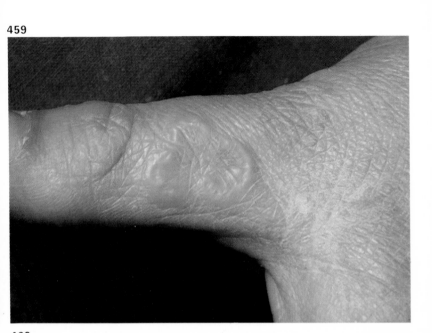

460

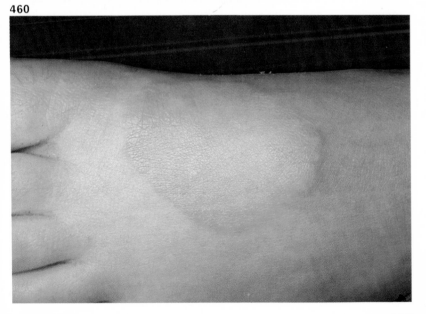

**461 *Lichen sclerosus et atrophicus ('white spot disease'),
perianal*** The affected skin is white and atrophic with a sharp margin.
It is more commonly found on the vulva where it is pruritic and potenti-
ally pre-cancerous. A good light is necessary to make the diagnosis
clinically. Scattered patches of the disease may be found also on the
trunk and limbs. This histology is characteristic.

462 *Balantis xerotica obliterans, penis* This is the male counter-
part of lichen sclerosus et atrophicus of the vulva. It is a rare cause of
phimosis and meatal stricture in the adult.

463 *Radiodermatitis, chronic, scalp* The patient had received an
overdose of radiation in the treatment of scalp ringworm when she was a
child. The result was an x-ray induced scarring alopecia. The features
are atrophy, telangiectasia, and variable pigmentary changes. After
several decades keratoses, and basal and squamous carcinomas may
arise.

461

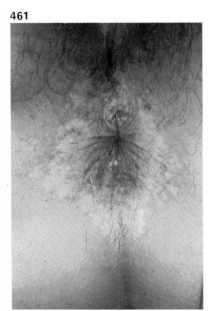

462

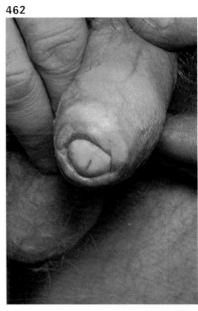

463

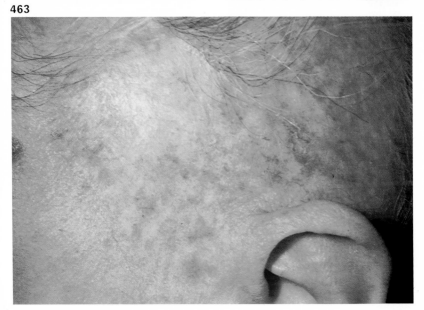

464 *Striae gravidarum, abdomen* Striae in pregnancy are so common as to be regarded as physiological. They may also be found around the hips and on the lower back and breasts. They are also common in both sexes at adolescence and in association with rapid weight gain. Striae are initially red or purple ; they eventually fade to leave thin silvery scars.

465 *Striae, steroid, thighs* The patient had applied an undiluted fluorinated steroid cream under polythene occlusion regularly for several months in the treatment of atopic dermatitis. Striae are also seen in Cushing's disease.

466 *Steroid erythema, face* The patient had applied undiluted topical fluorinated steroid ointment to the face every day for several months. A diffuse erythema is present. This complication is not seen when topical hydrocortisone preparations are used.

464

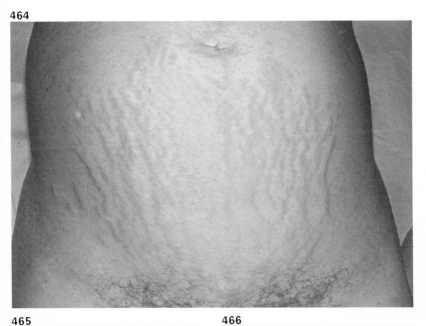

465

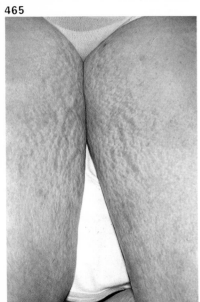

466

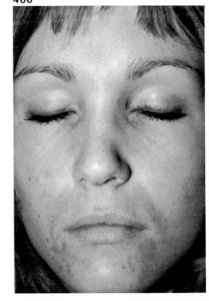

INDEX

FOR
REFERENCE ONLY

LEVENE, G M & CALNAN, C D
A colour atlas of dermatology

Please return/renew this item by the last date shown
Thank you for using your college library

SHEFFIELD COLLEGE - CASTLE CENTRE
Tel. 0114 260 2134